AN INTRODUCTION TO PARASITOLOGY

PHARMACEUTICAL MONOGRAPHS

GENERAL EDITOR

J. B. STENLAKE, D.Sc., Ph.D., F.P.S., F.R.I.C., F.R.S.E.

Professor of Pharmacy, University of Strathclyde

Volume 2

AN INTRODUCTION TO PARASITOLOGY

AN INTRODUCTION TO PARASITOLOGY

BY

JOHN M. WATSON

D.Sc. (London), A.R.C.Sc.

Principal Lecturer in Biology, West Ham College of Technology. Member of Expert Advisory Panel for Parasitic Diseases, World Health Organisation, Geneva

WILLIAM HEINEMANN MEDICAL BOOKS LTD

LONDON

First published 1965

Published by
Heinemann Medical Books Ltd
23 Bedford Square, London W.C.1

Printed in Great Britain by
Butler & Tanner Ltd, Frome and London

GENERAL PREFACE

The aim of this series of pharmaceutical monographs is to provide an up-to-date series of short publications for teaching general and specialised topics to undergraduate students of pharmacy and allied subjects. Each monograph in the series is the work of an expert or group of experts actively engaged in teaching or practice. A few of the introductory monographs are sufficiently comprehensive to warrant publication as individual volumes, but for convenience some of the shorter monographs on related subjects have been collected together for publication under one cover.

Each monograph is intended to serve as the basis for a group of lectures or tutorials in the honours and pre-honours years of undergraduate courses in pharmacy and allied subjects in British and Commonwealth Universities and, of necessity, some monographs are slanted towards the more specific requirements of these countries. We have, however, endeavoured to keep the monographs on a general plane to ensure their suitability for use in other parts of the world.

An attempt has been made to present the subject matter of individual monographs in such detail that it provides a permanent record for study purposes capable of being used by students in lieu of lecture notes. Each monograph, however, sets out to provide not merely a detailed account of essential subject matter, such as would be required for examination purposes, but also seeks to indicate its relevance and importance to pharmaceutical studies in general. In this respect the more advanced monographs extend naturally to the boundaries of knowledge in all major aspects, and wherever possible present appropriate rival views and hypotheses in sufficient detail for the student to grasp their essential detail without reference to the original. The texts are, however, referenced to provide additional sources of information.

I am indebted to the authors of the individual monographs for their willingness to collaborate with me in the preparation of this series. I should also like to express my thanks to my colleagues and many friends for their help and advice in framing the series and for discussions on individual monographs. I should further like to express my sincere thanks to Mrs S. Cohen for invaluable secretarial assistance.

J. B. S.

PREFACE TO VOLUME 2

Microbiological studies have long been emphasised in pharmaceutical education, particularly in so far as they reflect the requirement that injections shall be free from bacterial pathogens and the products of bacterial metabolism, and the need to protect an even wider range of pharmaceutical products from bacterial and mould contamination. Microbiological studies have also provided a firm foundation of knowledge for those concerned with the search for new agents and methods for combating bacteriological and viral infection. On the other hand, widespread interest in recent years in devising agents for combating other types of parasitic infection in humans and in animals has not been paralleled by any increase in the time devoted to the study of parasitology in undergraduate courses of pharmacy. The present volume, therefore, sets out to fill this gap by providing a text suitable for use by students of pharmacy and others interested in acquiring a more fundamental background of the various branches of animal parasitology. The study of protozoa (protozoology) and parasitic worms (helminthology) receive special attention as the prime agents of infection. Many insects act as intermediate hosts or mechanical vectors in the transmission of disease, and for this reason a chapter on entomology has also been included. An attempt has been made to classify and describe all the major parasites (other than those generally covered by the study of microbiology) responsible for disease in man and his domestic animals. The text includes descriptions of the major parasites, their hosts, intermediate hosts and vectors, and pathogenic effects, together with a brief description of agents and methods used in their control and elimination.

Although intended primarily to provide background information for courses of study in pharmacy, it is hoped that the text will find a wider sphere of usefulness as a text for those pursuing specialised courses in schools of human and veterinary medicine, and biology.

1964

J. M. W.

J. B. S.

CONTENTS

CHAPTER 1

INTRODUCTION

THE NATURE OF PARASITISM

Parasitism is a physiological association between two living organisms in which one associate (the *parasite*) has lost its physiological independence and relies upon the other associate (the *host*) for its nutritional requirements, and sometimes for other metabolic needs. The host not only receives no benefit in return but is often actively injured by the parasite.

Another form of physiological association between living organisms, known as *symbiosis*, is beneficial to both partners. Thus termites harbour certain species of flagellate protozoa in their alimentary canal, without the help of which they are unable to utilise the cellulose in their food and which, in turn, cannot live outside the termite gut.

All such physiological associations are necessarily of considerable duration; and may exist between animals, between plants, or between animals and plants. Long-term associations between living organisms of different species may, however, be ecological rather than physiological in nature. Thus, in *phoresis* one animal attaches itself to another animal in order to be carried from one place to another; while in *commensalism* each partner benefits ecologically from the activities of the other. An example of a phoretic association is supplied by the temnocephalid flatworms which attach themselves to large fresh water crustaceans, while commensalism is illustrated by the hermit crab *Eupagurus* which lives in association with the sea-anemone *Adamsia*, the crab benefiting from the protection afforded by the stinging cells of the anemone, which itself benefits by sharing the food of the crab.

CHARACTERISTICS OF PARASITES

Animal parasites, owing to their mode of life, have developed certain biological characters which distinguish them from other animals, as follows:

Physiological adaptation. This is illustrated by the ability of intestinal worms to adjust their respiratory processes to very low oxygen tensions and to resist the action of the digestive juices of the host.

Reduction or loss of organs. Sense organs, locomotor organs, specialised digestive organs and organs of predation, and other organs useful to a free-living animal but not to the sheltered parasite surrounded by its food and safe from attack by enemies, are frequently reduced or lacking.

Increased reproductive capacity. In order to compensate for the numerous adverse factors operating against the likelihood that the offspring will find and successfully invade new hosts and develop to maturity, reproductive capacity in parasitic forms is often much greater than in related free-living forms.

Modification of existing structures and development of new structures. The modification of the cuticle of intestinal worms to carry out selective absorption and the evolution of suckers, hooks and other organs of attachment are examples. Such organs are specifically useful in a parasitic existence.

Modification of the life history. In order to facilitate transmission from host to host the life history is often profoundly modified and may become very complex. In particular, reproduction by immature forms in order to facilitate production of offspring in large numbers, the adoption of intermediate and paratenic hosts, and the correlation of the life history of the parasite with the habits and life history of these and of the definitive host, may occur.

RELATIONSHIP OF PARASITES TO HOSTS

The relationship of an animal parasite to its host distinguishes it sharply from a predator, with which, since it subsists on other animals, it might otherwise be compared. The parasite must avoid killing the host, at any rate until there has been opportunity for its offspring to invade new hosts, since when the host dies the parasite dies with it. A predator, such as a tiger, on the other hand, destroys its prey rapidly and completely, since it remains free to seek other victims.

The detailed study of the whole range of interaction between parasite and host is sometimes included under the term **host-parasite relationships.**

KINDS OF PARASITES

Parasites are grouped biologically according to the nature of their relationship to the host and according to their type of life cycle, as follows.

Endoparasites and Ectoparasites

Endoparasites, such as hookworms, live inside the body of the host; whereas ectoparasites, such as fleas, attach themselves to the outside of the host's body.

Permanent and Temporary Parasites

Permanent parasites, such as tapeworms, spend the major part of their lives inside the host or, in some cases, attached to the surface of its body; whereas temporary parasites, such as mosquitoes, make contact with the host only from time to time, when it is necessary to feed.

Facultative and Obligate Parasites

Facultative parasites, such as *Rhabditis hominis*, are capable of leading either a parasitic or a free-living existence, according to circumstances; whereas obligate parasites, such as tapeworms, are incapable of continued existence away from the host.

Monoxenous, Heteroxenous and Autoheteroxenous Parasites

Monoxenous parasites, such as hookworms, require only a single host during each complete life cycle; heteroxenous parasites, such as tapeworms, need two or more different host species, namely a definitive host and one or more intermediate hosts, during each complete life cycle; while autoheteroxenous parasites, such as trichina worms, *Trichinella spiralis*, are those in which the definitive host of one generation becomes the intermediate host of the next generation.

Accidental Parasites

These are parasites that have entered unusual host species in which they can maintain themselves for a while, but not permanently. Thus the dog tapeworm, *Dipylidium caninum*, can establish itself for a while in man.

Spurious Parasites

These are free-living forms which have become accidentally introduced into a host and succeed in surviving therein for a time. Vinegar eels, *Turbatrix aceti*, introduced into the human vagina during douching, can maintain themselves there for a time.

THE BRANCHES OF PARASITOLOGY AND THE PLACE OF PARASITES IN THE ANIMAL AND PLANT KINGDOMS

The range of parasitic organisms which affect man and his domestic animals is so wide that it has become fragmented into several distinct disciplines, each dealing with the parasites belonging to a particular taxonomic group, as set out below.

(1) **Virology**

This is the study of the parasitic organisms known as the viruses, the majority of which are too small to be visible through the optical microscope.

(2) **Bacteriology**

This is the study of the members of the plant group Schizomycetes, closely allied to the Fungi.

(3) **Animal Parasitology**

This is the study of the parasitic members of the animal kingdom. It is often further subdivided as follows:

(*a*) *Protozoology*. This is the study of the members of the group Protozoa, and particularly of the parasitic members. These are minute unicellular animals, many of which are parasites.
(*b*) *Helminthology*. This is the study of the parasitic worms comprised within the following groups:
    Trematoda (flukes)
    Cestoda (tapeworms)
    Nematoda (roundworms)
    Acanthocephala (thorny-headed worms)
    Hirudinea (leeches).
(*c*) *Entomology*. Strictly speaking this is the study of insects in general, but, so far as parasitology is concerned, is usually understood to include the study of the parasitic members of

the animal phylum Arthropoda, which includes not only the insects but also the mites and ticks, spiders and other forms of medical and veterinary importance.

(4) **Mycology**

This is the study of the members of the plant group Fungi, a large number of which are parasitic.

Parasites occur in other groups of the animal and vegetable kingdoms but such forms are not of medical or veterinary importance.

PHYSIOLOGY OF PARASITES

Until quite recently very little was known about the physiological relationship between endoparasites and their hosts, but knowledge in this important field is now advancing rapidly. Experimental investigation requires efficient *in vitro* culture techniques, which are now being developed. Modern methods of investigation are being used to elucidate the composition of the body and its fluids; the nature of the food utilised and the processes of its assimilation; protein, fat and carbohydrate metabolism; respiratory processes; enzyme importance and reactions; excretion; osmotic relationships and tonicity; movement and locomotion; behaviour reactions; and growth. Much of this work is too recent to be seen in correct perspective against the dynamic background of the host–parasite relationship. Further consideration of these matters would be out of place in a monograph of the scope of the present work.

ECOLOGY OF PARASITES

The term 'ecology' includes the study of every aspect of the relationship between an organism and its environment. In the case of an endoparasite the host represents the environment and therefore host–parasite relationships really represent ecological problems of a special type, in which the physiology of both host and parasite plays a cardinal role. The consideration of such matters also lies outside the scope of the present work. However, many animal parasites have free-living stages in their life-history in order to facilitate transmision from one host to another; and these stages are affected by the external inanimate environment in much the same ways as any free-living animal. Development outside the host is influenced by many factors, but principally by temperature, moisture and oxygen supply. Not only survival but also speed of development of the free-living stages of parasites depends upon a favourable combination of these factors. Any excessive fluctuation in their level may retard development, or even be fatal; while climatic mean levels outside the favourable range will altogether prevent a parasite from establishing itself in a given area. Thus, although the eggs of human hookworms (q.v.) will hatch at any temperature between 7° C and 37° C, development is very slow below 15° C and the infective stage is not reached below 17° C; while temperatures outside the hatching range are sooner or later fatal to the free-living juveniles. The restriction of human hookworm infection to the warmer parts of the world and to mines in the temperate zones is due to the fact that the optimum temperature for the development of the free-living stages of this parasite lies between 23° C and 30° C; and where mean temperatures fall constantly outside these limits the worms will not be able to establish themselves. Humidity and oxygen tension similarly affect the free-living stages. Thus, free-living human hookworm juveniles cannot survive for long in soil which contains less than 9 per cent of water, and are rapidly destroyed by flooding. Hookworm eggs can only survive for just over a week in the complete absence of oxygen, and their development is retarded by micro-aerobic conditions. Free-living stages of other parasites show similar reactions to variation in these three major environmental factors. Light intensity, hydrogen-ion concentration, the nature of the soil or the composition of the water, and the presence or absence of vegetation are among the numerous ecological factors which influence the survival and development of the free-living stages of parasites.

LIFE-CYCLE OF PARASITES

Accurate knowledge of the life-cycle of a parasite is important in the design of effective and reliable diagnostic techniques, measures of prevention and control, and even treatment. To achieve these four aims it is necessary to know:

(1) The location of all stages of the parasite in or on the body of the definitive host.
(2) The way in which the parasite leaves the definitive host.
(3) The means by which it is transmitted to another definitive host.

(4) The means by which it gains entry to the new definitive host individual and the route followed within the body.
(5) The nature and environmental relationships of any free-living stages.
(6) The identity of any intermediate host (or hosts) and the ways in which the parasite infects it and leaves it again.
(7) Which of the stages of the whole life-cycle are most accessible and susceptible to attack, both within and without the body of the definitive host.

The majority of parasites have complex life-cycles and generalisation at this stage would be unwise. The life-cycle of each different group of parasitic forms is briefly summarised in later sections. Great variation exists, but in general it may be said that the life-cycles of parasites fall into two major groups.

(1) Those in which development is direct and no intermediate host is required, such as the dysentery amoeba, *Entamoeba histolytica*, and the human hookworm, *Ancylostoma duodenale*.

(2) Those in which development is indirect and one or more intermediate hosts are involved, within which larval or juvenile stages of the parasite must develop before becoming infective to the definitive or principal host. The intermediate host may be a mollusc (as in the case of the human blood flukes, *Schistosoma* spp.), or a blood-sucking insect (as in the case of the malaria parasites, *Plasmodium* spp.), a crustacean (as in the case of the Guinea worm, *Dracunculus medinensis*), or a vertebrate (as in the case of the beef tapeworm, *Taenia saginata*). Other animal groups are occasionally involved as intermediate hosts. Some parasites must pass through two different intermediate hosts in the course of one complete life-cycle as, for example, the human lung fluke, *Paragonimus westermani*, which infects first a water-snail and then a crustacean before reaching the adult stage in man.

Whether or not an **intermediate host** is involved, every parasite has a **principal or definitive host,** in or on which the mature adult stage is reached and sexual reproduction takes place. Animals, other than the normal definitive host species, in which the parasite can develop to the sexually mature stage are known as **reservoir hosts.**

INFECTION, TRANSMISSION AND DISSEMINATION OF PARASITES

The source of infection with any parasite is always an infected individual of one kind or another—definitive host, reservoir host or intermediate host. In the transfer of a parasite from one definitive host individual to another, three stages or operations are involved:

(1) The parasite must leave the first definitive host individual.
(2) It must then be transmitted to another definitive host individual.
(3) Finallly it must gain entry to the body of the new definitive host individual.

Failure in any of these three operations involves failure in transmission.

There are six principal avenues of exit from the body of the first definitive host individual.

(1) In the **faeces** (as the eggs of hookworms and tapeworms, and the cysts of dysentery amoebae).
(2) In the **urine** (as the eggs of the human blood-fluke, *Schistosoma haematobium*).
(3) In the **sputum** (as the eggs of lung-flukes and lung-worms).
(4) Through the **skin** (as the juveniles of the Guinea-worm, *Dracunculus medinensis*, which escape through a perforated cutaneous ulcer whenever this is submerged in water).
(5) In the **blood** (as the gamonts of malaria parasites and the microfilariae of Bancroft's filaria, which are removed by blood-sucking mosquitoes when feeding).
(6) Through **ingestion of the infected host** by another animal of the same or a different species (as the encysted juveniles of *Trichinella spiralis*).

Having escaped from the first definitive host individual the parasite must now be transmitted to a new definitive host individual by one of the following six agencies, depending on the species of parasite and the nature of its life-cycle.

(1) **Contact**—cysts of dysentery amoebae, eggs of the human threadworm, *Enterobius vermicularis*, and the pork tape-

worm, *Taenia solium*, may be transferred from faeces or the anus to the mouth on the fingers; and the mouth amoeba, *Entamoeba gingivalis*, is transferred from mouth to mouth by the act of kissing.

(2) **Food**—an agency particularly used by parasites of the digestive tract. In some cases flesh containing the infective stage of the parasite is eaten (as pork infected with larvae of the tapeworm, *Taenia solium*, or with juveniles of *Trichinella spiralis*); in others the infective stage of the parasite is attached to plants used for food (as encysted metacercariae of Busk's fluke, *Fasciolopsis buski*, to water chestnuts); in yet others vegetables or salads may be contaminated with faeces containing infective stages of a parasite (as salads contaminated with eggs of the roundworm, *Ascaris lumbricoides*).

(3) **Water**—which may contain infective eggs of various intestinal worms (as *Ascaris lumbricoides*), or cysts of intestinal protozoa (as dysentery amoebae), when used for drinking; or which may be a necessary medium for the passage of free-living stages (as the cercariae of blood-flukes).

(4) **Soil**—which may be contaminated with eggs or cysts of intestinal parasites (as whipworm eggs or amoebic cysts) or which may be the necessary medium in which an active infective stage develops (as in the case of human hookworms, the infective juveniles of which develop in soil and penetrate any human skin with which they come into contact).

(5) **Biological vectors or intermediate hosts**—as the blood-sucking mosquitoes which transmit malaria parasites and certain species of filarial worms.

(6) **Mechanical vectors**—i.e. insects such as house-flies which act as mechanical carriers of eggs of intestinal worms and cysts of intestinal protozoa from faeces to food, without being biologically involved in their life-cycles. Human beings with hands unwashed after defaecation can also act as mechanical vectors.

Having reached the new definitive host individual, the parasite must now invade it via one of the following avenues.

(1) **Direct contact**—as in the case of *Entamoeba gingivalis*, mentioned above.

(2) **Digestive tract**—i.e. by ingestion of food or water contaminated with the infective stages (hookworms, tapeworms, dysentery amoebae, etc.).

(3) **Skin**—i.e. active penetration by the infective stage of the parasite (juveniles of human hookworms, cercariae of blood-flukes).

(4) **Blood**—i.e. introduction of the infective stage of the parasite directly into the blood stream or into the lymph vessels by the bite of a blood-sucking insect, as in the case of malarial parasites and Bancroft's filaria.

HARMFUL EFFECTS OF PARASITES ON THE HOST

Parasites often produce harmful (pathogenic) effects upon their hosts which, naturally, are usually more marked in the case of endoparasites than in that of ectoparasites. The nature of these effects depends upon the avenue by which the parasite invades the host; upon the migration route in the case of those parasites which move from one location to another within the body of the host after infection; upon the final location of the adult parasite within the host body; upon the size and number of parasites present; and upon their activities within the host, especially their mode of feeding. The inimical effects which result fall into six principal categories as follows, although more than one of these may occur in any one infection.

(1) **Spoliative action**—as in the case of hookworms, which rob the host of blood, and of tapeworms, which deprive it of digested food.

(2) **Toxic action**—as in the case of malaria parasites, the poisonous metabolic by-products of which, liberated into the blood at intervals, are responsible for producing the characteristic febrile paroxysms of malaria.

(3) **Traumatic action**—as the damage to the muscular tissues caused by juveniles of *Trichinella spiralis* migrating to their encystment sites, and the damage to the wall of the colon caused by invading dysentery amoebae.

(4) **Mechanical action**—as the pressure effects produced by large hydatid cysts and the blockage of the bile duct or pancreatic duct sometimes produced by wandering individuals of *Ascaris lumbricoides*.

(5) **Irritative and inflammatory action**—as the duodenal irritation caused by *Giardia lamblia*, the characteristic rise in the eosinophil count which occurs in many helminthic diseases, and the fibrosis which is typically produced around the eggs or immobilised juveniles and adult stages of parasitic worms embedded in the tissues.

(6) **Secondary effects**—as the weakening of the resistance of the host to other infections, and the bacterial invasion of lesions in tissues and organs initially produced by animal parasites.

The nature of the pathogenic effects varies with the stage of the parasitic infection, and will be different during the invasion phase, the incubation and migration phases, the active phase and the chronic phase of the disease. Characteristic lesions are usually caused by each different species of parasite in particular organs of the host; and symptoms vary accordingly. Further information is given under each species of parasite (below).

RESISTANCE AND IMMUNITY TO PARASITIC INFECTIONS

The host is rarely a passive victim of any parasite. It manifests complete **natural resistance** or immunity (basic or innate immunity) to all those parasite species which are unable to establish themselves in or on it. Thus, dog fleas do not survive long on man; and any given species of tapeworm can generally establish itself successfully in only one or, at most, a few closely related, species of host. This restriction of a species of parasite to one host species or to a small number of closely related forms is known as **host specificity.** It finds its explanation in the very close correspondence which must exist between the physiological needs of the parasite and the physiological environment which the host can provide; and the phenomenon of natural immunity has therefore, in general, a physiological basis.

Once invaded by a species of parasite to which it is susceptible however, the host soon begins to defend itself actively, a process known as the development of **acquired immunity**; and there ensues a fluctuating balance between the invasiveness of the parasite and the defences of the host. The result of acquired immunity in parasitic diseases, unlike that in bacterial diseases, is usually not the complete elimination or destruction of the invading organism, but a restriction of its numbers, activity, growth-rate and fertility. The stimulus which results in the development of acquired immunity consists in the presence in the host tissues of alien chemical substances of high molecular weight, known as **antigens,** produced by the parasite. The resulting effects fall into two groups.

Humoral Response

As a result of the stimulation of the reticulo-endothelial system by the antigens, specific substances known as **antibodies** are produced. An antibody generally reacts with, and only with, the antigen which provoked its formation; but occasionally a single antigen may incite the formation of a spectrum of antibodies, which may react with a whole series of substances related chemically to the antigen. The **antigen–antibody reaction** is believed to be a physical rather than a chemical phenomenon; it invariably leads to fixation of a thermolabile constituent of the blood serum known as the **complement (alexin)**; and may be followed by any of the following phenomena.

(*a*) **Agglutination** or clumping of particulate antigens or antigen-containing organisms, which may occur with very small parasites.
(*b*) **Precipitation** of a soluble antigen by its specific antibody.
(*c*) **Lysis,** i.e. the killing and dissolution of the antigenic organism by the combined action of antibodies and complement.
(*d*) **Neutralization** of toxins by antitoxins.

There are differences between humoral response to parasitic invasion and humoral response to bacterial or viral invasion; but these appear to be differences of degree rather than of kind. For instance, **toxin–antitoxin reactions** are of less frequent occurrence in parasitic infections, owing to the fact that true **exotoxins** are less often produced by animal parasites than by bacteria and viruses.[1]

Cellular Response

In many parasitic infections protective activities on the part of the white cells of the blood, lymph glands and vasoformative tissues, and on the part of fibroblasts, are not only more pronounced than humoral response, but are also more conspicuous

[1] **Antitoxins** are a special form of antibody produced in response to the stimulus of a toxic antigen, with which they react to neutralise it.

than in the majority of viral and bacterial infections. **Macrophages** operate singly against very small parasites in the same way that they do against bacteria. Large parasites, once they have been immobilised in the tissues, are attacked by vast armies of macrophages, and often demolished piecemeal (as blood-flukes immobilised in the liver or lungs). **Eosinophil cells,** always produced in larger numbers in parasitic infections, are believed to play an important role in the detoxification of parasite proteins and their disintegration products. Connective tissue cells, especially **fibroblasts**, are important in walling-off parasites and enclosing them within fibrous capsules—often the ultimate phase in their immobilisation, which enables the macrophages to attack them successfully.

Acquired immunity to parasitic, as to bacterial and viral, infections, exists in two forms, namely, **residual immunity** and **tolerance immunity (premunition)**. In a few protozoal infections (such as cutaneous leishmaniasis) the immune response may be powerful enough not only to destroy the invading organisms but also to render further infection impossible. In the majority of parasitic infections, however, premunition is the rule, the immune response being relatively weak and depending for its continuance on the continued antigenic stimulation exerted by the restricted parasite population.

Many hosts show **age resistance** to particular parasites; but the mechanism of this phenomenon varies from species to species and cannot be discussed here. Hosts frequently show remarkable tolerance to the injurious effects of parasites, often owing to stimulation and increased efficiency of tissue repair mechanisms.

Artificial immunisation against parasitic infections has not passed beyond the experimental stage, so far as man is concerned; although a form of immunisation against the cattle lung-worm, *Dictyocaulus*, is now successfully practised. Considerable use of immune reactions in parasitic infections is made in connection with diagnosis, a variety of serological tests being regularly employed.

GEOGRAPHICAL DISTRIBUTION OF PARASITIC INFECTIONS

Parasites are obviously limited geographically primarily by the distribution of their principal or definitive and reservoir hosts. Distribution of intermediate hosts may, however, also be a limiting factor, as in the case of the three species of human blood-flukes, which only occur where the appropriate water-snails are found. Climatic conditions may also exert a limiting influence, as in the case of human hookworm disease already mentioned above. The customs and habits of the human host may also affect the presence or absence of specific parasitic infections in particular localities. Thus, trichinelliasis and pork tapeworm infection are conspicuously absent in Moslem countries, owing to the fact that the inhabitants abstain from eating any form of pork or pork products. In Europe and North America, high levels of hygiene and sanitation have very largely eliminated ascariasis. Parasitic infections in which no host other than man is required, or in which there is an intermediate or reservoir host of cosmopolitan distribution, and in which there are no vulnerable free-living stages, are necessarily of world-wide distribution. Such infections are exemplified by the human thread-worm.

In the case of certain human parasitic diseases known as **zoonoses,** distribution is complicated by the fact that the disease is common to man and certain species of lower mammals, which maintain the infection in areas where it might be otherwise eliminated in the human population. Zoonoses are, of course, really infections in which the reservoir hosts are of paramount importance. Among important zoonoses may be mentioned hydatid disease and cutaneous leishmaniasis.

Nomenclature of Parasitic Infections

The nomenclature of parasitic infections is generally derived from the root of the generic name of the parasite, with the addition of the suffix '-iasis'. Thus infection with *Ancylostoma duodenale* is termed ancylostomiasis, and infection with any species of parasitic amoeba is termed amoebiasis. The termination '-osis' is, however, sanctioned by tradition or euphony in certain cases. Thus infection with *Toxoplasma* spp. is termed toxoplasmosis, and infection with *Trichostrongylus* spp. is termed trichostrongylosis. A few diseases have popular names which are in general use, such as malaria and hookworm disease. A somewhat artificial distinction is often maintained between symptomless cases of light infection with a parasite and cases of heavy infection in which disease is patent; but this is only a matter of degree.

CHAPTER 2

PROTOZOOLOGY

NATURE AND CLASSIFICATION OF PROTOZOA

The phylum Protozoa includes the simplest and most primitive members of the animal kingdom. The organisms of which it is composed are characteristically unicellular (or non-cellular), multiply by fission, and show no parent body after reproduction. Most form protective cysts by means of which dispersal or transmission is effected. They are divided into four distinct groups on the basis of their nuclear apparatus and locomotor mechanism.

(1) **Sarcodina**

These are amoeboid forms moving by means of pseudopodia and lacking a pellicle. The nucleus is single. Most are free-living but some are parasitic, notably species of the genera *Entamoeba*, *Dientamoeba*, *Endolimax* and *Iodamoeba*.

(2) **Mastigophora**

These are flagellate forms moving by means of one or more long whip-like structures (flagella) arising from and controlled by a basal apparatus. They possess a pellicle. The nucleus is single. Most are free-living but some are parasitic, notably members of the genera *Giardia*, *Trichomonas*, *Trypanosoma*, *Leishmania*, *Hexamita* and *Histomonas*.

(3) **Ciliophora**

These are ciliated forms moving by means of a series of integrated rows of short hair-like structures (cilia) controlled by a complex neuromotor apparatus. A pellicle is present. Many have a cell-mouth or cytostome and show elaborate morphological differentiation within the cell. Most have two nuclei—a macronucleus which governs the vegetative functions (feeding, movement, respiration, excretion, etc.) and a micronucleus which controls conjugation and reproduction; but a small number have numerous nuclei. Most are free-living, but some are parasitic, notably members of the sub-class Protociliata (*Opalina et al.*), of the group Entodiniomorpha (*Entodinium et al.*) and of the genus *Balantidium*.

(4) **Sporozoa**

All the members of this group are parasitic and lack any specialised locomotor mechanism. Unlike the other groups there is generally a complex life-cycle. The nuclear arrangement varies with the stage of development. Important genera from the medical and veterinary point of view are *Plasmodium*, *Haemoproteus*, *Leucocytozoon*, *Babesia*, *Theileria*, *Anaplasma*, *Isospora*, *Eimeria*, *Toxoplasma* and *Sarcocystis*.

SARCODINA

(AMOEBAE)

The Dysentery Amoeba (*Entamoeba histolytica*)

This is the most important amoeboid parasite of man. It is cosmopolitan in distribution but is more prevalent in warm climates than in the temperate zones. Disease symptoms occur in a relatively small proportion (10 per cent) of infected persons, owing to the existence of strains or races of varying virulence.

There are three stages in the life-cycle.

(1) The active, motile, typically amoeboid, tissue-invading stage, which is 20 to 30 microns in diameter. It is known as the trophozoite.
(2) The smaller, more sluggish pre-cystic stage, which is 7 to 18 microns in diameter.
(3) The spherical, resistant, tough-walled cyst—5 to 20 microns in diameter—which is characterised by possessing four nuclei and a glycogen body. It passes out of the host in the faeces.

Transmission is by ingestion of food or water contaminated with cysts from the faeces of an infected person. The cysts hatch in the small intestine, giving rise to small amoebae which, after division, develop into trophozoites in the colon.

Non-virulent races live in the lumen of the colon and do no harm to the host; but virulent races invade the mucosa of the colon by means of cytolytic ferments and give rise to small, flask-shaped abscesses, which may enlarge and coalesce to form crateriform ulcers. Deep abscesses may permit the amoebae to reach blood vessels and to be carried by the blood stream to the liver, where they multiply and set up further abscesses in the hepatic tissue.

The infection is normally chronic and mild or symptomless; but virulent strains or races of the parasite may cause an acute syndrome in persons whose resistance is low and in whom the intestinal ulcers become secondarily infected with pyogenic bacteria. Abdominal discomfort or pain, and diarrhoea or dysentery are the usual symptoms in such cases. Amoebic liver abscess is characterised by fever, tenderness and enlargement of the liver, and dull pain generally referred to the right shoulder.

Diagnosis is by finding the characteristic cysts in the faeces.

A variety of specifics have been used in treatment, notably emetine, various organic compounds of iodine and arsenic, and, recently, various antibiotics.

Preventive measures involve sanitary disposal of sewage and human excrement; boiling or filtration and hyperchlorination of drinking water (normal chlorination alone is not sufficient to kill the cysts); thorough washing of salads and vegetables, especially if they have been fertilized with night-soil; elimination of the infection in carriers, especially food-handlers; anti-fly measures, since these insects carry the cysts on their feet and in their gut from faeces to food; and personal hygiene, especially the washing of hands after defaecation and before eating.

Other Amoebae Parasitic in Man

Several cosmopolitan species of amoeba are parasitic in man, in addition to *E. histolytica*, but normally none of them invade the mucosa and so they do not usually cause disease:

Entamoeba coli. This species occurs in the large intestine of man and resembles *E. histolytica*, with only minor differences, in morphology and life-cycle. It is never pathogenic.

Entamoeba gingivalis. This species occurs in the human mouth, and also resembles *E. histolytica.* It lacks a cystic stage, however, and is transmitted by direct contact, droplet spray, or contaminated dishes or vessels.

Endolimax nana. This is a smaller form with oval cysts which also occurs in the large intestine, both of man and of monkeys.

Iodamoeba butschlii. This is another small form with irregularly shaped cysts. It occurs in the intestine of man and pig, and is rarer than the preceding forms. Fatal cases of generalised infection with this species have been reported.

Dientamoeba fragilis. This is a relatively rare form occurring in the large intestine of man. It is still smaller than the two preceding species and has, apparently, no cystic stage. The mode of transmission is unknown. Some workers have believed that it may produce a syndrome characterised by nausea, vomiting, diarrhoea and abdominal pain.

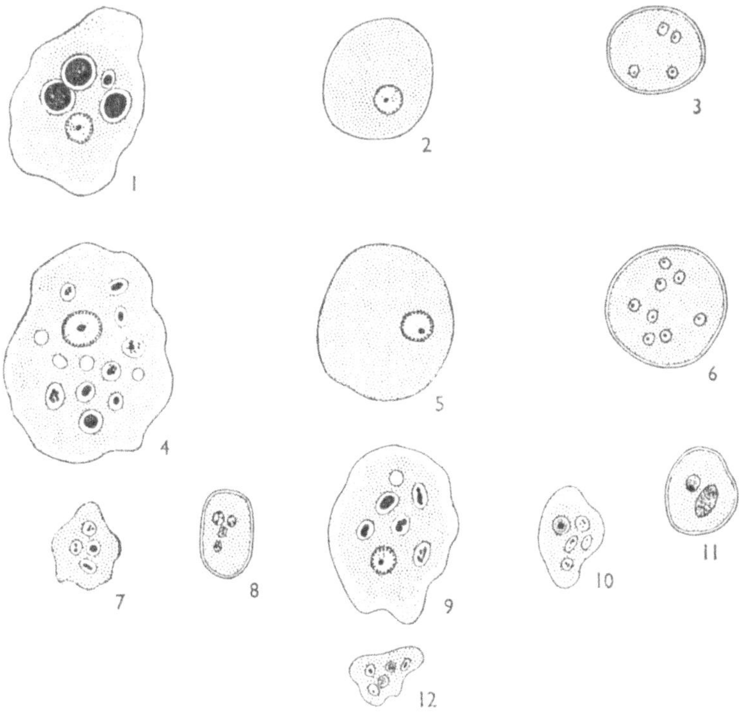

FIG. 1

1 *Entamoeba histolytica*—trophozoite from lesion in intestinal wall, showing erythrocytes in course of digestion.
2 —precystic form.
3 —cyst.
4 *Entamoeba coli*—trophozoite.
5 —precystic form.
6 —cyst.
7 *Endolimax nana*—trophozoite.
8 —cyst.
9 *Entamoeba gingivalis*—trophozoite.
10 *Iodamoeba bütschlii*—trophozoite.
11 —cyst.
12 *Dientamoeba fragilis*.

These various species of human amoebae are readily differentiated under the microscope by the shape and size of the cysts through which transmission is achieved, and by the structure of their nuclei.

Amoebae Parasitic in Domestic Animals

A number of different kinds of amoebae, including not only species of *Entamoeba* but also *E. histolytica* itself, occur commonly in domestic animals. None of them, however, are normally of pathogenic importance.

MASTIGOPHORA (FLAGELLATES)

Intestinal and Oral Parasites of Man

Giardia lamblia. This cosmopolitan species is the only flagellate parasite of the human alimentary tract which shows undisputed pathogenicity. There are two stages in the life-cycle, the trophozoite and the cyst.

The **trophozoite** is a small (10–21 by 5–15 microns) pear-shaped organism with a convex dorsal surface and a flat ventral surface provided with a large oval sucker. It lives in the small intestine, especially the duodenum, attached to the mucosa by means of its sucker; but can move in a jerky, actively progressive way through the agency of four pairs of flagella, namely, anterior and middle pairs arising from the anterior basal bodies, a ventral pair arising from the axostyles, and a caudal pair arising from the posterior basal bodies, The two pairs of basal bodies connected by the axostyles constitute the controlling neuromotor apparatus. There is a pair of ovoid nuclei.

The **cyst** is a small (8–12 by 7–10 microns) ovoid body.

Transmission is effected in the same way as in *E. histolytica*. Infection is often symptomless, especially in adults, since the parasite does not invade the tissues; but irritation and inflammation of the mucosa may be caused by the sucking discs, with resulting chronic mucous diarrhoea, upper abdominal pain, anorexia and loss of weight. Children are more frequently infected than adults especially in institutions and may show retardation of growth.

Diagnosis is by finding the characteristic cysts in the faeces or in the duodenal drainage. Acranil and mepacrine are both specific, the infection clearing up rapidly after treatment. Prevention involves the same measures as for *E. histolytica* infection.

Other Flagellates Parasitic in the Human Alimentary Tract

The following species are all non-pathogenic, but pathological conditions of the intestine due to other agents, especially those causing diarrhoea, probably favour their multiplication and discharge in the faeces. This has sometimes led to the erroneous conclusion that they were themselves the etiological agents.

(*a*) *Trichomonas hominis.*
(*b*) *Enteromonas hominis.*
(*c*) *Chilomastix mesnili.*
(*d*) *Embadomonas intestinalis.*

All four species are small, cosmopolitan forms with characteristic numbers and arrangement of flagellae. They are transmitted by means of characteristically shaped cysts, with the exception of *T. hominis*, which apparently has no cystic stage but possesses a very resistant trophozoite.

Another form with no cystic stage—*Trichomonas buccalis*—occurs in the human mouth and is transmitted, like *E. gingivalis*, by direct contact, droplet spray, or contaminated dishes or vessels.

Vaginal Parasites of Man

Trichomonas vaginalis is a small cosmopolitan species which occurs in the vaginal secretions of woman and occasionally in the urethral discharges of man. In women it is often associated with vaginitis, urethritis and leucorrhoea, but some doubt exists as to whether it is always the etiological agent. In man it is apparently non-pathogenic. Transmission probably occurs during intercourse. Diagnosis is by finding the parasite in the appropriate secretions. Treatment varies according to the view taken of its pathogenicity. There is no practical method of prevention.

Blood Parasites of Man

The flagellate parasites of the human blood stream are very small, actively motile forms belonging to the genus *Trypanosoma*. The body is elongate, the nucleus central, and the basal apparatus situated at the posterior end. A single flagellum arising from the basal apparatus extends forwards along the side of the body, to which it is connected by an undulating membrane, and projects freely at the anterior end. Short, broad forms without a flagellum also occur. The life-cycle involves a blood-sucking intermediate host, within which further multiplication takes place. Three species are common parasites of man.

T. gambiense. This species is widely distributed in Africa between the parallels of 15° N and 15° S. It is transmitted by tsetse-flies (*Glossina palpalis* usually but *G. tachinoides* in some areas) which ingest infected blood from man and within which the parasite develops and multiplies before being injected into a new definitive host when the fly bites again. Domestic and wild animals of various kinds are believed by some authorities to act as reservoir hosts. In the early stages of the disease, when the trypanosomes are in the blood and lymph, there is irregular intermittent fever, soon followed by lymphatic enlargement as the lymph glands are invaded. Later the parasites reach the cerebrospinal fluid and bone marrow, and the classical syndrome of sleeping sickness develops, characterised by anaemia, headache and aching pains in the back and limbs, by constant hectic fever, and by increasing mental dullness, languor and apathy. Drowsiness increases and the patient becomes comatose and emaciated, and finally succumbs. Death is usually due to secondary infection. Diagnosis is by finding the trypanosomes in the blood, lymph gland extract, bone marrow or cerebrospinal fluid. Treatment, usually with organic arsenicals or Suramin (Bayer 205), must be commenced early to be effective. Prevention involves anti-tsetse-fly measures, protection from tsetse bites, control of population movements in infected areas, and removal of the human population from hyper-endemic regions.

T. rhodesiense. This species is similar to *T. gambiense*, but occurs in East Africa and is transmitted by *G. morsitans*. Wild game animals are believed to act as reservoir hosts. The disease produced in man is essentially the same as that produced by *T. gambiense*, but is more acute and runs a more rapid course.

T. cruzi. This species occurs in South America, especially Brazil, and is transmitted by *Triatoma megista* and other blood-sucking reduviid bugs. When feeding these insects deposit a drop of infected faeces which the host may inoculate into the wound by scratching. Many species of wild and domestic animals act as reservoir hosts. The parasites invade and multiply in the tissues, especially the cells of the reticulo-endothelial system, the neuroglia cells of the central nervous system and the heart muscle cells, producing aflagellate 'leishmania' forms. The principal lesions are usually in the heart wall, brain and liver. In the acute form of the disease there is fever, oedema of the eyes and face, adenitis, anaemia, and myocarditis which may be fatal. In non-fatal cases infection subsides in a few weeks and a chronic condition develops which may persist for years, with symptoms varying according to the location of the parasites. In the early stages diagnosis is by examination of blood-smears for the trypanosomes, while in the later stages animal inoculation, **xenodiagnosis** (feeding a healthy bug on the blood of the suspected individual and subsequently examining it for the parasite) or immunological tests must be used. There is no effective treatment for this infection. Prevention is by destruction of the insect vectors and protection from their bites.

Tissue Parasites of Man

The flagellate parasites of human tissues are very small (2–5 microns) ovoid, intracellular forms belonging to the genus *Leishmania* and transmitted by blood-sucking sand-flies (*Phlebotomus* spp.). The stage in man (Leishman-Donovan bodies) occurs in the spleen or in the skin and elsewhere in the reticulo-endothelial system; and lacks a flagellum. Larger (14–20 microns), motile, flagellate forms develop in the gut of the intermediate host and are injected when it bites another human being. Dogs and gerbils may be naturally infected and act as reservoir hosts. Three distinct syndromes are produced but the life-cycles are similar and the parasites morphologically indistinguishable in each. Physiological differences justify the erection of three species.

Kala-azar (*L. donovani*). This syndrome occurs in the Mediterranean region, Central and North Africa, and Central and Southern Asia. The parasites principally occur in the liver and spleen but may also infect other parts of the reticulo-endothelial system, especially the bone marrow and macrophages in the lymph glands of the intestine, which ulcerate. There are two distinct varieties of kala-azar, depending upon whether the infection is with the adult or infantile strain.

In the **adult form** periods of high fever with rigors alternate with periods of apyrexia for months, ultimately culminating in continuous low fever with progressive splenomegaly, anaemia, leucopenia, emaciation, and a characteristic earthy grey colour of the skin. Untreated cases usually terminate fatally due to exhaustion or inter-current disease.

In the **infantile form** there is irregular fever, progressive anaemia, mental delusion, emaciation, abdominal distension, progressive splenomegaly, purpuric haemorrhages and cachexia. Spontaneous recovery occasionally occurs, otherwise death from complications takes place within three years. Recovery is followed by life-long immunity.

Diagnosis involves demonstration of the parasite by microscopical examination of peripheral blood films, spleen-, liver- or bone-marrow-puncture material; by culture of peripheral blood or nasal secretions; or by animal inoculation of material. Special immunological tests also exist. Pentavalent antimonials and diamidines are used in treatment. Prevention involves anti-sand-fly measures and protection from their bites; destruction of dogs (reservoir hosts) and isolation of cases.

Oriental sore (*L. tropica*). This syndrome has an essentially similar distribution to kala-azar, although it does not extend so far east and shows other local variations. The infection is confined to the skin around the bite of the infected intermediate host, where an itching, sharp-edged, shallow ulcer develops from an initial papule and discharges a thin watery fluid. There are no systemic symptoms. Healing occurs naturally but slowly after many months. Two types of ulcer are observed, namely, a dry type characteristic of towns, in which the papule does not ulcerate for months, and a moist or wet type characteristic of desert settlements and rural areas in which the papule ulcerates at once. The wet type is a zoonosis affecting chiefly gerbils. Immunity for life results from one attack, but no cross-immunity exists between the wet and dry types. Diagnosis is by finding the parasite in material extracted from the margin of the sore with a Pasteur pipette. Treatment, other than prevention or cure of secondary infection, is not essential; but trivalent and pentavalent antimonials are used systemically, and more rapid healing has been claimed to follow a variety of local applications. Prevention involves principally anti-sand-fly measures and protection from bites; destruction of reservoir hosts (gerbils and dogs) has also been recommended.

Espundia (*L. braziliensis*). This syndrome is also known as **American muco-cutaneous leishmaniasis.** It occurs in Central and Southern America. The first sign of the disease is a cutaneous ulcer resembling Oriental sore, usually on the face. In a proportion of cases the infection extends onto mucous surfaces, leading to the development of fungating and eroding ulcers of the tongue and the linings of the buccal and nasal cavities. Lymph glands, but not the internal organs, may also be affected. The cutaneous ulcers heal but the mucous lesions persist and gradually become more

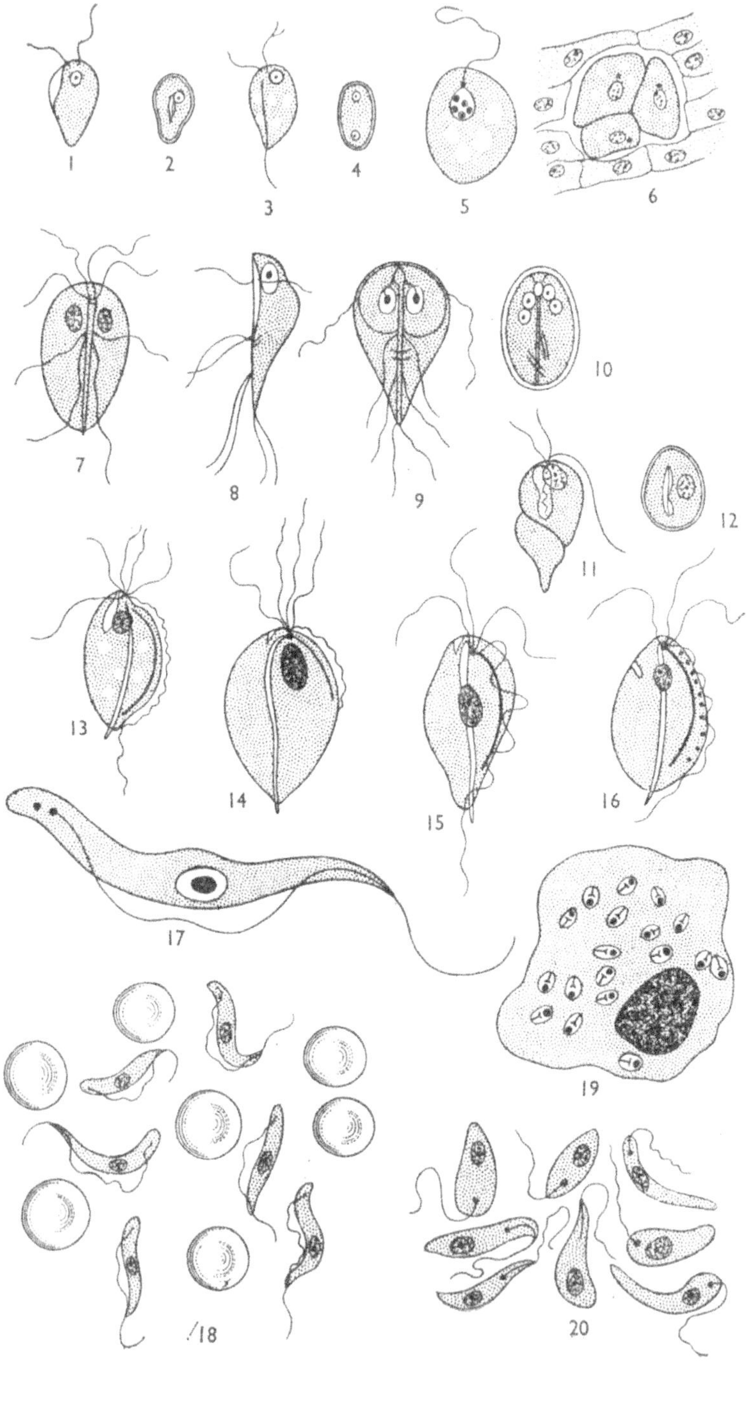
1
2
3
4
5
6
7
8
9
10
11
12
13
14
15
16
17
18
19
20

extensive. Local pain, fever and anaemia are concurrent symptoms. Death may occur due to complications. Like kala-azar and oriental sore this is an endemic disease, but reaches epidemic proportions when human beings go into the forest for lumber and other purposes. It most frequently affects children and young adult males. Diagnosis is by finding the parasite in scrapings or puncture material from lesions, and by immunological tests. Treatment in the cutaneous stage is similar to that for oriental sore. Once mucosal lesions have developed, local infiltration of atebrine solution and intravenous or intramuscular injections of antimonials may be used. Antibiotics are necessary against secondary infection. Prevention involves anti-sand-fly measures and protection from their bites.

Flagellate Parasites of Domestic Animals

Trichomonas foetalis occurs in the vagina of cows causing inflammation which may result in early abortion and even in sterility. Cows develop immunity but the bulls which transmit the infection do not do so.

Trichomonas gallinae occurs in the small intestine and liver of turkeys, producing serious lesions and causing a severe and often fatal condition characterised by diarrhoea.

Hexamita meleagridis also occurs in the intestine of turkeys, causing a severe and often fatal form of enteritis.

Histomonas meleagridis occurs in both intestine and liver of poultry and game-birds, causing a form of enterohepatitis known as blackhead disease. This condition is mild in chickens but very

---

FIG. 2

1 *Embadomonas intestinalis*—trophozoite.
2 —cyst.
3 *Enteromonas hominis*—trophozoite.
4 —cyst.
5 *Histomonas meleagridis*—flagellate form from culture.
6 —aflagellate trophozoites in a liver-lesion.
7 *Hexamita meleagridis*.
8 *Giardia lamblia*—trophozoite in side view.
9 —trophozoite from above.
10 —cyst.
11 *Chilomastix mesnili*—trophozoite.
12 —cyst.
13 *Trichomonas hominis*.
14 *Trichomonas vaginalis*.
15 *Trichomonas foetalis*.
16 *Trichomonas gallinarum*.
17 *Typical trypanosome*.
18 *Trypanosoma gambiense* in blood of host.
19 *Leishmania donovani*—aflagellate forms in an endothelial cell.
20 *Leishmania tropica*—flagellate forms from culture.

severe in turkeys. Transmission is by direct contamination of food, as with other intestinal parasites, but can also occur by introduction of the parasite with the eggs of the nematode worm *Heterakis gallinae*.

A number of other species of intestinal flagellates occur in domestic animals, but none of them are proven pathogens.

Species of the genus *Trypanosoma* cause severe disease in the larger domestic animals in the warmer parts of the world, as shown in Table 1.

TABLE 1

Parasite	Usual definitive host	Disease	Vector	Comment
T. equiperdum	Horses	Dourine	None. Transmitted during sexual intercourse via genital abrasions	Fatal in stallions; less severe in mares. South Europe, Asia, Africa, North America
T. evansi	Horses, cattle, camels	Surra	Horse-flies, tabanids and other blood-sucking flies	Virulence varies—many strains. In warm countries throughout the world
T. brucei	Cattle, sheep, goats, pigs, horses, camels, dogs	Nagana	Tsetse-flies (*G. morsitans*)	Sometimes fatal in domestic animals—symptomless in wild ungulates. Tropical Africa
T. vivax	Cattle, sheep, goats, horses	Souma	Tsetse-flies or tabanids	Sometimes fatal in domestic animals—symptomless in antelopes. Africa, West Indies, Central and South America
T. equinum	Horses	Mal de Caderas	Tabanids	South America
T. congolense	Horses cattle, sheep, goats, pigs	—	Tsetse-flies	Severity in domestic animals varies—antelopes symptomless carriers. Tropical Africa
T. simiae	Pigs, monkeys	—	Tsetse-flies or tabanids	Highly pathogenic. Tropical Africa
T. theileri	Cattle	—	Tabanids	All parts of the world

CILIOPHORA
(CILIATES)

Balantidium coli. This cosmopolitan species is a parasite of pigs and monkeys, which relatively rarely infects man. It is a large (50–100 microns by 40–70 microns), actively motile form having an antero-lateral peristome leading in to a cystostome. It inhabits the lumen of the large intestine, but frequently invades and damages the intestinal wall. Large (45–65 microns), highly resistant, spherical or ovoid cysts are formed and pass out in the faeces of the host. Transmission is as in *Entamoeba histolytica.* Man is usually resistant to

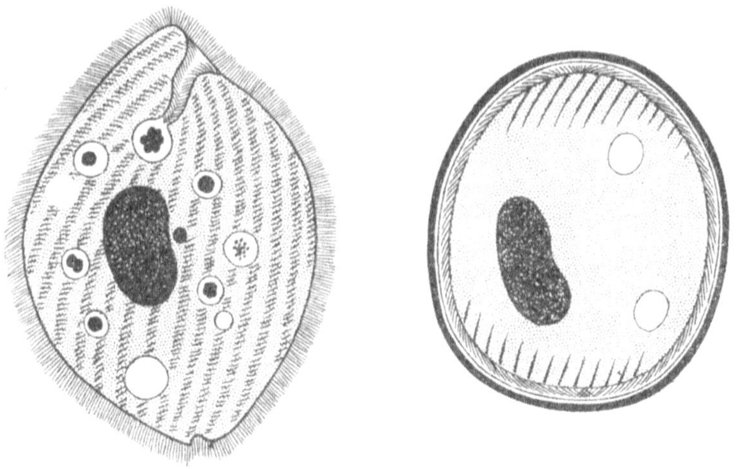

FIG. 3

Balantidum coli
Trophozoite

Balantidum coli
Cyst

cross-infection with this parasite from the normal host—the pig; but once infection has been established in man it is easily transmitted to other human beings. Extensive abscess formation and ulceration may occur in the mucosa and submucosa of the large intestine, and secondary infection may develop. Some cases are symptomless, but usually there is diarrhoea or dysentery with abdominal tenderness or pain and nausea or vomiting. Anorexia, headache and insomnia may develop. Diagnosis is by finding the active ciliates or their cysts in the faeces. Many treatments have been recommended but none has proved to be specific.

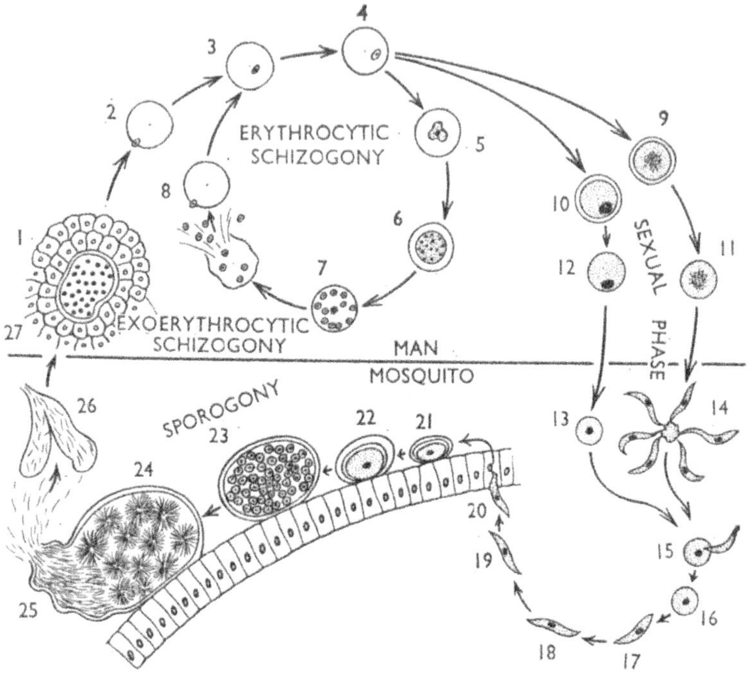

1
2
3
4
5
6
7
8
9
10
11
12
13
14
15
16
17
18
19
20
21
22
23
24
25
26
27
ERYTHROCYTIC SCHIZOGONY
EXOERYTHROCYTIC SCHIZOGONY
SEXUAL PHASE
MAN
MOSQUITO
SPOROGONY

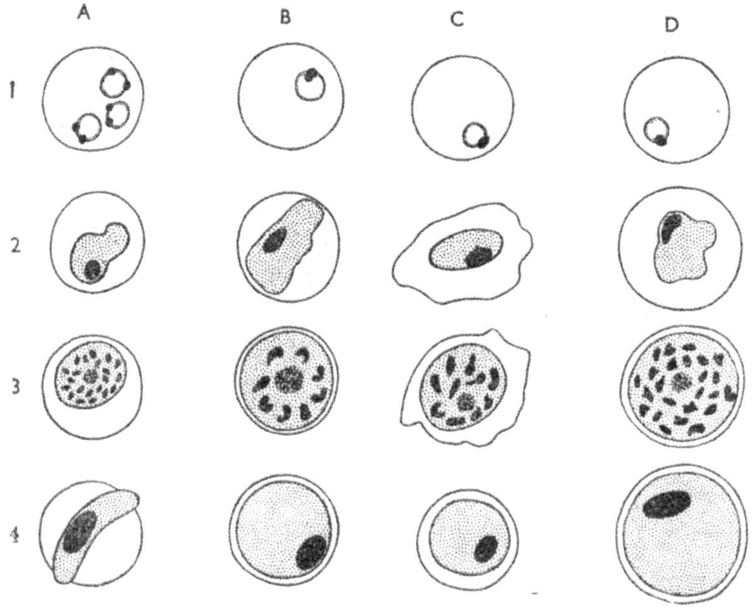

A
B
C
D
1
2
3
4

Spontaneous cure may occur. Prevention involves personal cleanliness and avoidance of contact with pigs.

There are no other important ciliate parasites of man or domestic animals. *B. coli* in pigs is apparently harmless.

SPOROZOA

Malaria Parasites (*Plasmodium spp.*)

The following species of this genus are the most important sporozoan parasites of man:

P. malariae which causes quartan malaria (characterised by a febrile paroxysm every 72 hours).

FIG. 4. Malaria Parasites

Upper figure—Life-cycle of *Plasmodium* spp.

Erythrocytic cycle (Schizogony):
1 Exo-erythrocytic stage in liver—schizogony.
2 Merozoite entering erythrocyte.
3 Ring form (very young trophozoite).
4 Young trophozoite.
5 Half-grown trophozoite.
6 Segmenting form—first stage of schizogony.
7 Segmented form—schizogony completed.
8 Merozoite entering erythrocyte.

Sexual cycle:
9 Male gametocyte in erythrocyte.
10 Female gametocyte in erythrocyte.
11 Male gametocyte free in plasma.
12 Female gametocyte free in plasma.
13 Male gametes forming from male gametocyte.
14 Female gamete formed from female gametocyte.
15 Fertilisation taking place.
16 Zygote.

Sporogony,
17 Oökinete.
18 Oökinete }
19 Oökinete } making its way to epithelial cell of mosquito stomach wall.
20 Oökinete penetrating epithelial cell.
21 Oöcyst forming on outer side of stomach wall.
22 Oöcyst enlarging.
23 Sporoblasts forming inside cyst.
24 Sporozoites forming by division of sporoblasts and escaping by bursting of cyst.
25 Sporozoites making their way through haemocoele to salivary gland.
26 Sporozoites in salivary gland of mosquito.
27 Sporozoites entering liver of human host.

N.B.—Stages 1 to 12 and 27 in man (primary host).
Stages 13 to 26 in mosquito (secondary host).

Lower figure—Comparative Features of Human Malaria Parasites in Blood.

A *Plasmodium falciparum.*
B *Plasmodium malariae.*
C *Plasmodium ovale.*
D *Plasmodium vivax.*

1 Ring stages.
2 Trophozoites.
3 Segmenting forms.
4 Gametocytes.

P. vivax and *P. ovale* which cause benign tertian malaria (characterised by a febrile paroxysm every 48 hours).

P. falciparum which causes malignant (pernicious) tertian malaria (characterised by febrile paroxysms at irregular intervals approximating to 48 hours in some cases).

The life-cycle of all four species is essentially similar. It involves certain mosquito species belonging to the genus *Anopheles* as intermediate hosts, and passes through four stages:

(*a*) the pre-erythrocytic cycle
(*b*) the exo-erythrocytic cycle
(*c*) the erythrocytic cycle
(*d*) the sexual cycle.

(1) **The pre-erythrocytic cycle.** When a human being is bitten by an infected mosquito, the slender, motile **sporozoites** of the parasite are injected into the blood stream, which they leave within an hour to invade the liver. Here they enter the parenchymatous cells and grow rapidly to form **schizozoites** which divide (**schizogony**) to form a large number of small **merozoites**.

(2) **The exo-erythrocytic cycle.** The majority of the merozoites emerge into the blood-stream and invade red blood corpuscles, but some may re-infect liver cells and form a reservoir of infection in the liver .

(3) **The erythrocytic cycle.** Those merozoites which invade erythrocytes feed on their contents and grow into **trophozoites**, each of which divides to form a further generation of merozoites (**schizogony**). Each daughter merozoite invades a further erythrocyte.

(4) **The sexual cycle** begins in man and is completed in the mosquito. Instead of developing into trophozoites and undergoing division, the merozoites grow into more compact cells known as **gamonts** or **gametocytes**, of which two kinds may be distinguished —the male or **microgametocyte** and the female or **megagametocyte**. The gametocytes undergo no further development unless they are ingested by an appropriate species of mosquito, when they are liberated by digestion from the enveloping corpuscle and divide to form elongate, motile male gametes or rounded passive female gametes, according to their sex. Male and female gametes unite to form **zygotes**, which become motile and penetrate epithelial cells of the stomach wall. Between the epithelial and subepithelial layers

each zygote becomes enclosed in a cyst and divides repeatedly therein to form a large number of minute, vermiform, actively motile **sporozoites**. Eventually the cyst bursts and the sporozoites are liberated into the haemocoele or body cavity of the mosquito, through which they make their way forwards to the salivary glands, there to lie in wait for an opportunity to invade a new human host when the infected mosquito bites again.

In addition to the typical paroxysms, involving fever and rigor, which coincide with the bursting of infected erythrocytes and the discharge of merozoites and toxic metabolic by-products into the blood plasma, malaria is characterised by anaemia (resulting from destruction of red blood corpuscles) and by enlargement of the spleen. Paroxysms recur regularly in untreated cases until immunity builds up to the level at which it can impose latency on the parasite. In malignant malaria the fever is remittent not intermittent, and all the symptoms are more severe. Headache is often pronounced in all forms of malarial fever.

Diagnosis is by finding the parasites in films of the peripheral blood. Considerable skill and experience are required to differentiate the various species of *Plasmodium* in each stage of the life-cycle. Some of the principal differences are given in Table 2.

Until the last quarter century the classical drug used in treatment was quinine, but atebrine (mepacrine, quinacrine) was then discovered to be specific. It has since been joined by plasmoquine (pamaquine), chloroquin (aralen diphosphate), paludrine (chlorguanide) and daraprim (pyrimethamine). These drugs differ in their efficiency against the different stages and species of the parasite.

Malaria formerly killed millions of human beings every year and is still the most important single disease in warm climates, especially Asia, Africa and Southern Europe. It was introduced into America by European colonists and African slaves. Its incidence, prevalence and severity are affected directly or indirectly by a large number of factors including race, age, sex, occupation, locality, climate, season, soil, altitude, humidity and immunity.

Prevention involves anti-mosquito measures and mass chemotherapy of human populations in endemic areas. The relatively recent introduction of insecticides effective against the vectors, and of new and more effective drugs for use in treatment, together with a world-wide campaign against the disease directed and co-ordinated by the World Health Organisation have done much to reduce the ravages of malaria in the last fifteen years.

TABLE 2

Stage	*P. malariae*	*P. vivax*	*P. ovale*	*P. falciparum*
Very young trophozoite—ring form (see footnote 1)	One nucleus	One nucleus	One nucleus	Two nuclei
Growing trophozoite (schizont)	Motility slight. Band-shaped	Actively amoeboid until half-grown	Motility slight. Form ovoid	Actively amoeboid throughout
Mature trophozoite (schizont)	Occupies all of infected erythrocyte	Occupies all of infected erythrocyte	Occupies three-quarters of infected erythrocyte	Occupies two-thirds to three-quarters of infected erythrocyte
Infected erythrocyte	Normal shape and size	Normal shape but much enlarged; and with Schüffner's dots (see footnote 2)	Irregular shape; slightly enlarged; and with Schüffner's dots	Normal shape and size but with Maurer's dots (see footnote 3)
	Multiple infection very rare	Multiple infection common	Multiple infection rare	Multiple infection very common
	Contains coarse granules of dark brown or black pigment	Contains fine granules of yellow-brown pigment	Contains coarse granules of dark brown or black pigment	Contains coarse granules of dark brown or black pigment
Division (schizogony, segmentation)	Dividing forms oval, round or band-shaped	Dividing forms irregular	Dividing forms oval or round	Dividing forms not seen in peripheral blood
	Merozoites—6–12 (8–10 usually)	Merozoites—12–24 (18–20 usually)	Merozoites—6–12	Merozoites 8–36 (18–24 usually)
	Central mass of pigment—symmetrical arrangement	Irregularly round central pigment mass	Round central or excentric pigment mass	Central pigment mass
Gametocytes	Round—fill infected erythrocyte	Round—fill infected erythrocyte	Round—but only three-quarters fill infected erythrocyte	Crescent- or kidney-shaped; free in blood plasma

(1) *Ring form*—the very young intra-corpuscular trophozoite, so-called on account of the 'signet ring' appearance caused by the large central vacuole and protuberant lateral nucleus.

(2) *Schüffner's dots*—fine, round, pink, eosinophilic granules.

(3) *Maurer's dots*—irregular dark-red spots or clefts in the cytoplasm, perhaps representing cytoplasmic precipitates.

Other Sporozoa Parasitic in Man

Isospora hominis. This is a widely distributed but relatively uncommon parasite of man in temperate climates. It inhabits the small intestine and forms small (20–33 by 10–19 microns), elongate-ovoid **oöcysts** with a smooth two-layered wall, which pass out in the faeces. The parasite within the oöcyst divides to form two **sporoblasts**, each of which secretes a cyst-wall around itself and divides therein to produce four, long, slender **sporozoites**. If the oöcysts are ingested by a fresh host, the sporozoites emerge on reaching the ileum and invade cells of the epithelial lining. Here they develop into **trophozoites** and divide (**schizogony**), giving rise to **merozoites** which invade other epithelial cells. Eventually a sexual phase supervenes, **macro-** and **micro-gametes** being formed from **gametocytes** and uniting to form **zygotes**, each of which secretes an oöcyst around itself. Transmission is by ingestion of faecal-contaminated material, as in the case of *Entamoeba histolytica*, there being no intermediate host. The rarity of the infection in man implies the existence of a reservoir host; but this has not so far been identified. Many cases are symptomless, but in some there is a short, mild, self-terminating diarrhoea, accompanied by anorexia, nausea and abdominal pain. Diagnosis is by identification of the characteristic oöcysts in the faeces. There is no specific treatment. Prevention is by the same measures that are used against *E. histolytica* infection.

Toxoplasma gondii. This is a small (4–6 by 2–3 microns), elongate, crescent-shaped, uninucleate organism, occurring in endothelial cells. It is widely distributed in man, and is much commoner than was formerly supposed. It is probably identical with species occurring in lower mammals. The symptoms in man vary according to the location of the parasites, so that the following principal forms of the disease have come to be recognised.

Congenital type—parasites in the brain—mental and psychomotor symptoms.

Meningo-encephalitic type—parasites in the brain and spinal cord—encephalitic symptoms.

Generalised type—parasites in the lungs (pneumonia), myocardium (myocarditis), liver, spleen, bone-marrow, adrenal glands, lymph glands, kidneys and nervous system (mental symptoms and encephalitis)—high fever and skin eruption, diverse other symptoms.

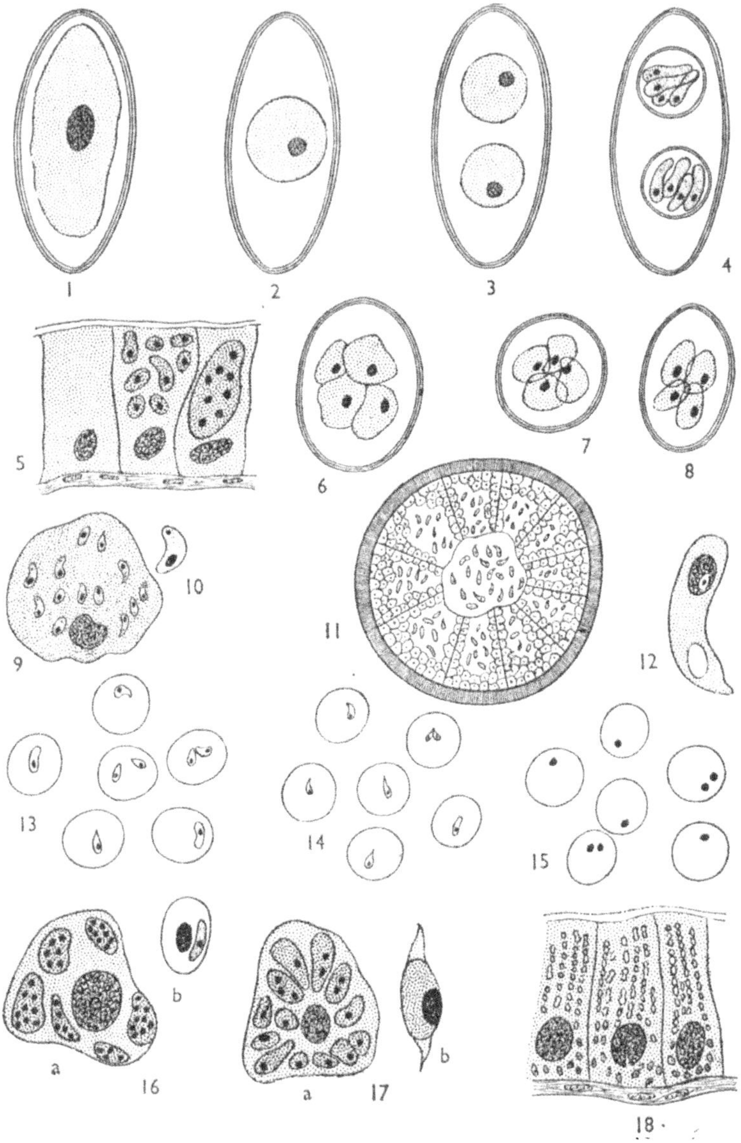

FIG. 5

1 *Isospora hominis* oöcyst—unsporulated.
2 —prior to formation of sporoblasts.
3 —with two sporoblasts.
4 —with two spores each containing four sporozoites.
5 *I. felis*—mature schizont and merozoites in epithelial cells of intestine of cat.
6 *Eimeria tenella*—oöcyst.

Symptomless type—especially in infected mothers who may give birth to infected children.

Infection can be fatal, especially in children. Transmission is either congenital (to the foetus *in utero* or to the offspring via the milk), or from external sources (probably by droplet infection, contaminated food or tick bite). Diagnosis is by isolation of the organism from infected tissues or body fluids, or by immunological tests. Antibiotics, antiserum and sulfa drugs have been used in treatment.

Sarcocystis lindemanni. This is a rare tissue parasite of man, morphologically indistinguishable from species occurring in lower mammals. It inhabits the intestinal wall and the muscles of the heart, larynx, tongue and extremities. Elongate **sarcocysts (Miescher's tubes)**, ranging from a few microns up to several centimetres in length, are found among the muscle fibres, each divided by septa into chambers containing rounded cells that give rise to bean-shaped **spores (Rainey's corpuscles)**, rounded at one end and pointed at the other. When the cyst is ingested by a suitable host the spores are liberated, penetrate epithelial cells of the intestinal wall, and multiply by binary fission. The daughters enter the lymph and blood corpuscles of the villi and are carried to the muscles, where they develop into new sarcocysts. The symptoms of sarcosporidiosis are not well defined; but heavy infections may cause death, owing to the secretion by the parasites of a potent toxin—sarcocystin. Diagnosis usually only takes place after death. There is no treatment. Prevention involves avoiding ingestion of uncooked meat.

Sporozoa of Veterinary Importance

A large number of species belonging to this group cause disease in domestic animals.

Haemoproteus malariae causes malaria in pigeons.

---

7 *Eimeria zurnii*—spherical oöcyst.
8 —ellipsoidal oöcyst.
9 *Toxoplasma gondii*—individuals in an endothelial cell.
10 —single.
11 *Sarcocystis lindemanni*—diagrammatic transverse section of Miescher's tube.
12 —Rainey's corpuscle (spore).
13 *Babesia bigemina* in erythrocytes of cattle.
14 *Theileria parva* in erythrocytes of cattle.
15 *Anaplasma marginale* in erythrocytes of cattle.
16 *Haemoproteus columbae*—multinucleate schizonts in endothelial cell of pigeon (a).
—developing female gametocyte in red blood corpuscle (b).
17 *Leucocytozoon anatis*—schizonts in endothelial cell (a).
—female gametocyte in distorted reticulocyte (b).
18 *Nosema bombycis*—dividing meronts (schizonts) in intestinal epithelial cells of silkworm (*Bombyx mori*).

Leucocytozoon anatis in ducks and *L. smithi* in turkeys cause a serious malarial syndrome marked by debility and death in non-immune young birds.

Piroplasms are minute non-pigmented parasites of the blood-cells, transmitted cyclically by hard ticks. The following are important:

Babesia bigemina causes red-water fever (Texas cattle fever) in cattle in warm climates. *B. bovis* causes a similar syndrome in temperate climates. *B. equi* and *B. caballi* cause biliary fever in horses. Other species cause malignant jaundice in dogs, pigs, sheep and goats.

Theileria parva causes East Coast cattle fever and *T. dispar* causes Mediterranean cattle fever. Another species of this genus occurs in sheep.

Anaplasma spp. cause gall-sickness of cattle, sheep and goats.

Several species of *Isospora* occur in dogs and cats.

A number of species belonging to the genus *Eimeria* are common parasites of live-stock. They are similar in morphology and life-cycle to *Isospora hominis*, but the oöcysts contain four sporocysts each of which contains two sporozoites. Infection with these forms is known as coccidiosis. *E. zurnii* causes the fatal disease of cattle known as red diarrhoea and several other pathogenic species occur in bovines. *E. arloingi* and several other species cause coccidiosis in sheep and goats. *E. debliecki* is one of several species pathogenic in young pigs. *E. perforans*, *E. magna* and *E. stiedae* affect rabbits and may damage the liver. Of the eight species parasitic in poultry, two—*E. tenella* and *E. necatrix*—are seriously pathogenic, the former in particular being responsible for heavy losses in young birds. *Tyzzeria perniciosa* causes coccidiosis in ducks in the U.S.A. Among other treatments, sulphonamides have been successfully used. Prevention involves keeping young animals in clean, dry conditions and avoiding over-crowding. Infection followed by recovery confers lasting immunity.

Toxoplasma spp., probably identical with *T. gondii*, cause a fatal syndrome in pigeons, sheep and, more rarely, other domestic animals.

Sarcocystis spp., probably identical with *S. lindemanni*, are pathogenic in domestic animals and poultry.

Nosema bombycis causes pébrine in honey bees.

CHAPTER 3

HELMINTHOLOGY

NATURE AND CLASSIFICATION OF PARASITIC WORMS

Helminthology is the study of parasitic worms. The word 'worm' has no exact zoological meaning, but includes all those invertebrate animals which have an elongate body without appendages and, often, without having a clearly differentiated head-region. In parasitic worms, the outermost layer of the body is usually a selectively permeable cuticle.

Parasitic worms are found in several groups of the animal kingdom.

Platyhelminthes (Flatworms)

This phylum includes dorsoventrally flattened worms in which a body-cavity is lacking, the space between the body-wall and the wall of the alimentary canal being filled with loose parenchymatous tissue. Excretion is by means of flame-cells. The majority are hermaphrodite and possess very complex genitalia. Parasitic forms are provided with special organs for attachment to the host. The group includes a free-living class **Turbellaria (Planarians),** and two parasitic classes which have evolved therefrom.

(*a*) **Trematoda (Flukes).** The majority are leaf-shaped animals with no segmentation, real or apparent; anterior and postero-ventral organs of attachment, which are usually suckers; and an alimentary canal generally consisting of a muscular pharynx and a blind intestine which may be a simple sac or consist of two caeca, often with diverticula. There is a complex life-cycle involving one or more intermediate hosts, the first of which is always a snail. The adults may be gut or tissue parasites of the definitive host. The larvae are always tissue parasites of the secondary host (or hosts.)

(*b*) **Cestoidea.** Most, but not all, the members of this class are segmented but not metameric worms known as **tapeworms.** The body consists of a terminal **scolex** or organ of attachment and a series of segments or **proglottides** known collectively as the **strobila.** The scolex is provided with suckers or adhesive outgrowths, and often with hooks as well; and is normally buried in the intestinal mucosa of the definitive host. Each proglottide contains one or more sets of reproductive organs. Young proglottides are produced by budding from the neck of the scolex; and mature proglottides full of ripe eggs are therefore found at the opposite end of the body. There is no alimentary canal, nutriment being absorbed through the surface of the body. The life-cycle is complex, involving at least one intermediate host. The adult worms are always intestinal parasites of the definitive host, while the immature stages are always tissue parasites of the intermediate host. Transmission is by ingestion of the infected intermediate host by the definitive host, either as food or by accident.

Acanthocephala (Thorny-headed Worms)

The members of this small phylum have an elongate, cylindrical body provided with a **retractile proboscis** armed by recurved hooks. An alimentary canal is lacking, nutriment being absorbed through the surface of the body. The sexes are separate. The life-cycle is complex, involving one or more intermediate hosts. The adult worms are intestinal parasites of vertebrate definitive hosts which become infected by ingesting the arthropod intermediate hosts in which the larval forms occur.

Nematoda (Roundworms)

The nematodes form a large and important class of the phylum Aschelminthes, the members of which have a straight gut and a non-coelomic body cavity or **pseudocoel.** This phylum also includes such forms as the rotifers. Many species of nematodes are free-living, some are plant parasites, and a considerable number are parasitic in animal hosts. They are unsegmented worms without suckers, having a cylindrical body which usually tapers at both ends. The straight, simple alimentary canal has an anterior mouth opening and a ventral, subterminal anus. The sexes are separate. The immature stages, generally known as larvae, are more correctly termed **juveniles,** since they differ from the adult only in their smaller size and lesser degree of differentiation. The life-cycle is exceedingly varied, ranging from direct and simple to very complex, indirect types. This large class is divided into upwards of twenty orders, only half of which include animal-parasitic species.

Hirudinea (Leeches)

Leeches belong to the phylum Annelida, the members of which have a long, metamerically segmented body; a coelomic body-cavity; a straight digestive tract with terminal mouth and anus; and, except in leeches, paired bristles or chaetae. The leeches are aquatic or terrestrial worms with large terminal suckers for locomotion and attachment. Some species are active predators, others are parasitic. The coelomic cavity is largely occluded by connective tissue and muscle. The individuals are hermaphrodite; the eggs are laid in cocoons; and the young, on hatching, resemble the parents except for their smaller size and sexual immaturity.

BIOLOGY OF PARASITIC WORMS

Parasitic worms do not multiply inside the body of the definitive host, but produce eggs or juveniles which must leave the host body before they can become adult[1]. Hence they all have to spend part of the life-cycle outside the definitive host before they can become infective again. Some are free-living during this period, while others require one or more intermediate hosts in which to continue their development. In the latter case the geographical distribution of the intermediate host or hosts limits that of the parasite just as it does in the case of malaria or other insect-transmitted protozoan diseases.

Development outside the body of the definitive host generally falls into one of the following categories:

(1) The unhatched eggs lie about on the ground and become infective after a time, as in the case of *Ascaris lumbricoides* and *Enterobius vermicularis* (q.v.).
(2) The eggs hatch on the ground and give rise to free-living juvenile forms which live in the soil and eventually become infective, as in the case of the human hookworms.
(3) The eggs hatch after or before leaving the definitive host and give rise to free-living juveniles which establish themselves in an intermediate host, as in the case of the Guinea Worm, *Dracunculus medinensis*, and the species of the genus *Schistosoma*.

[1] The only exception is the small nematode *Probstmayria vivipara*, which multiplies in the colon of horses and other equines.

(4) The eggs lie about on the ground and are swallowed by an intermediate host; as in the case of the majority of tapeworm species.
(5) The eggs hatch in the body of the definitive host and the juveniles are ingested with the blood or lymph of the host by a blood-sucking vector, usually an insect; as in the case of the various species of filarial worms.
(6) The eggs hatch in the body of the definitive host and the juveniles encyst therein and are ingested along with the host itself by another definitive host individual; as in the case of *Trichinella spiralis.*

Infective stages of parasitic helminths employ three channels of entry into the body of the definitive host, as follows:

(1) By ingestion through the mouth in food or drink; as in the case of *Ascaris lumbricoides*, *Enterobius vermicularis*, *Dracunculus medinensis*, *Fasciolopsis buski* and the various species of tapeworms.
(2) By direct invasion through the skin, as in the case of the hookworms *Ancylostoma duodenale* and *Necator americanus* and the various species of the genus *Schistosoma.*
(3) By injection through the skin into the tissues, blood or lymph by the agency of a blood-sucking intermediate host, as in the case of the various filarial worms.

Most helminths which enter the body of the definitive host in food or drink (and some which do not, such as the human hookworms) are intestinal parasites; but some migrate to other sites. Thus *Clonorchis sinensis* lodges in the bile-ducts and *Paragonimus westermani* eventually settles in the lungs.

PATHOGENIC EFFECTS OF PARASITIC WORMS

All parasitic worms rob the host of food materials in some way—either by absorbing digested food from the intestine, as do intestinal roundworms and adult tapeworms; or by sucking blood, as do hookworms; or by ingesting blood corpuscles, as do schistosomes; or by absorbing blood plasma or lymph, as do filarial worms; or by ingesting mucus and tissue cells, as do the liver flukes.

Local reaction may be slight, but some worms (such as the

schistosomes) cause extensive damage to the host tissues, while others (such as *Ascaris lumbricoides* and *Wuchereria bancrofti*) cause obstruction by blocking the lumen of essential organs like the intestine, the pancreatic duct or the lymph vessels; while yet others (such as *Fasciola hepatica*) induce tissue hypertrophy. Fibrosis and eosinophilia are characteristic host reactions to invasion of the tissues by parasitic worms. Toxaemia may occur to a variable extent.

Symptoms and pathogenic effects due to the young stages may be as serious as those due to the adult parasites. Thus the juveniles of *Ascaris lumbricoides*, migrating through the lungs, may cause a fatal pneumonitis and the condition known as hydatid cyst is caused by the larvae of the dog tapeworm *Echinococcus granulosus*.

However, infected persons, whatever the stage of the parasite, often show no symptoms, especially in light infections. They are, nevertheless, a source of infection to others and, as such, of public health importance.

TREMATODA

(FLUKES)

General

The Trematoda are divided into three sub-classes known as the Monogenea, the Aspidobothria and the Digenea. The members of the two first-named sub-classes are ecto- or endoparasites of cold-blooded vertebrates or higher invertebrates; and have a simple life-cycle with no alternation of hosts. The forms of importance in human and veterinary medicine all belong to the third group, the members of which are all endoparasitic species with a complex life-cycle involving several larval stages and at least one intermediate host. The organs of attachment in the Digenea consist of muscular anterior and ventral suckers, the former usually surrounding the mouth and therefore often known as the oral sucker. The adult fluke occurs in the body of the definitive host. The eggs escape in the faeces, urine or sputum; and hatch in water or after being ingested by the molluscan first intermediate host, liberating a ciliated larval form known as the **miracidium.** In most cases the miracidium swims freely in the water and actively penetrates the skin or gut-wall of the snail intermediate host, within which it develops into the second larval form or **sporocyst.** This gives rise parthogenetically to a number of individuals of the third larval stage or **redia.** Each redia, in turn, then gives rise by further parthenogenesis either to a second generation of rediae or to the fourth larval stage, known as the **cercaria.** This last-named form escapes

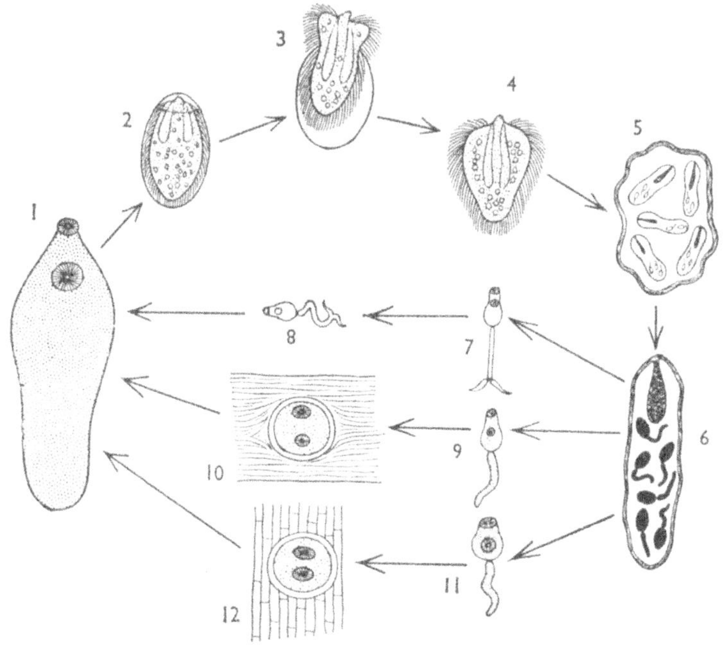

FIG. 6. Life-cycle of Trematoda (generalised)

1 Adult fluke (in definitive host).
2 Egg (passes out in faeces, urine or sputum).
3 Egg hatching (usually in water).
4 Miracidium (usually free-swimming in water and penetrates or is swallowed by first intermediate host).
5 Sporocyst containing rediae (in first intermediate host).
6 Redia containing cercariae (in first intermediate host).
7/8 Cercaria type I (free-swimming—seeks and penetrates definitive host).
9/10 Cercaria type II (free-swimming—seeks and encysts in second intermediate host, which is subsequently ingested by definitive host).
11/12 Cercaria type III (free-swimming—encysts on aquatic or submerged vegetation which is subsequently ingested by definitive host).

from the first intermediate host, which is generally an amphibious or aquatic snail, and swims freely in the water by means of its powerful muscular tail, seeking either the definitive host which it will penetrate directly (schistosomes) or a suitable encystment site. The latter may be a second intermediate host, or a plant, which must be ingested by the definitive host if the life-cycle is to continue.

The final infective stage, migrating within the body of the definitive host or enclosed within the cyst, is known as a **metacercaria.** When it reaches the appropriate location in the body of the definitive host it develops a reproductive system and transforms itself into an adult fluke.

Intestinal Trematodes

The following trematode species infect the human alimentary tract.

Gastrodiscoides hominis. This is a medium-sized (5 by 10 mm) fluke which occurs in India and parts of South-East Asia and attaches itself to the wall of the caecum and ascending colon, producing mucous diarrhoea. The life-cycle is unknown, but a related form occurring in horses (*Gastrodiscus aegyptiacus*) utilises species of the snail genus *Cleopatra* as intermediate hosts, the cercariae encysting on vegetation. Man probably acquires the infection by ingesting encysted metacercariae on uncooked vegetables or salads or in water. The pig is a reservoir host.

Fasciolopsis buski (**Busk's fluke**). This large (8–20 by 20–75 mm) elongate-ovoid fluke is common and widely distributed in the Far East, especially South-East Asia and Central and South China. It inhabits the upper part of the small intestine, attached to the wall, where it provokes ulceration of the mucosa, interferes with the secretion of the digestive juices and causes severe toxaemia resulting in abdominal pain, generalised oedema, diarrhoea, anorexia, nausea, vomiting and flatulence. Snails of the genera *Segmentina* and *Hippeutis* are utilised as intermediate hosts, the cercariae encysting on aquatic vegetation. Man acquires the infection by ingesting the cercariae on water chestnuts (*Eliocharis tuberosa*) and other aquatic salad vegetables when eating them raw or peeling them with the teeth. The pig is an important reservoir host.

Heterophyes heterophyes (**Dwarf fluke of man**). This is a small (1–2 by 3–4 mm) fluke common in the Nile Delta and in foci in the Far East. It occurs attached to the wall of the jejunum and upper ileum, where it provokes mild inflammation resulting in colicky pains and mucous diarrhoea. The infection is self-terminating in about two months. In Egypt the intermediate host is the snail *Pirenella conica*, while in China and Japan *Cerithidia cingulata* fills this role. On emergence from the snail the cercariae penetrate under the scales of various species of fresh-water fish and encyst in the superficial musculature. Man acquires the infection by eating

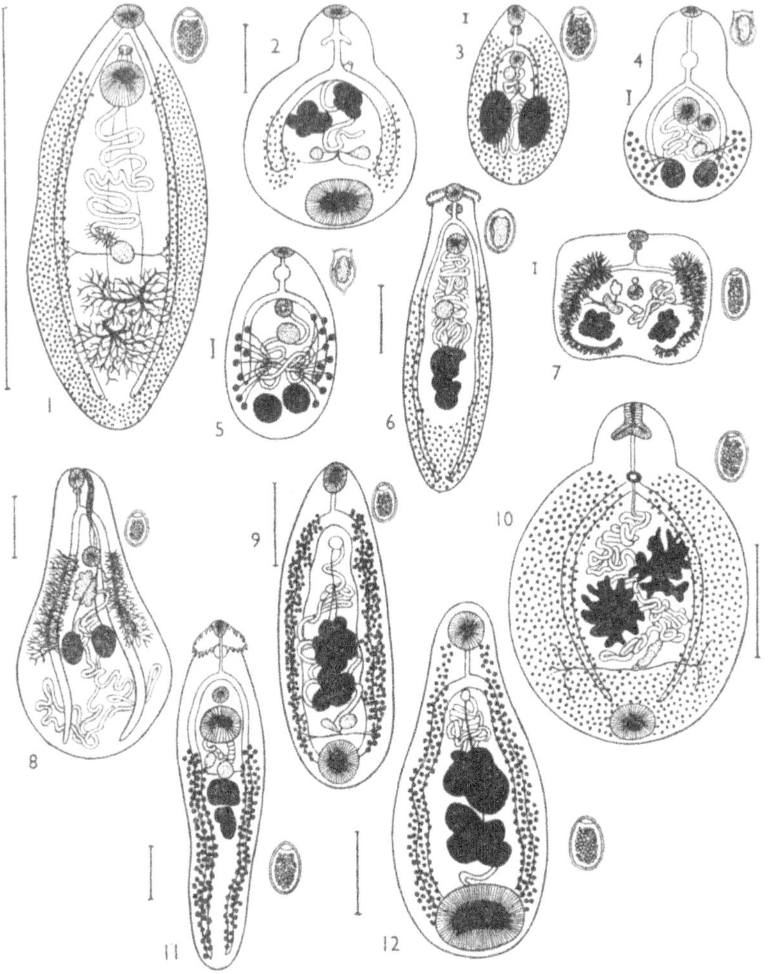

FIG. 7

Gut Flukes (Intestinal Trematodes) of Man and their eggs

1 *Fasciolopsis buski.*
2 *Gastrodiscoides hominis.*
3 *Troglotrema salmincola.*
4 *Heterophyes heterophyes.*
5 *Metagonimus yokogawai.*
6 *Echinostomum ilocanum.*

Gut Flukes (Intestinal Trematodes) of Domestic Animals and their eggs

7 *Euryhelmis squamula.*
8 *Prosthogonimus pellucidus.*
9 *Cotylophoron cotylophorum.*
10 *Gastrodiscus aegyptiacus.*
11 *Euparyphium melis.*
12 *Paramphistomum cervi.*

N.B.—Line beside each drawing indicates actual length of fluke.

infected raw or under-cooked fish. Dogs, cats, foxes and other fish-eating mammals are reservoir hosts.

Metagonimus yokogawai (**Yokogawa's fluke**). This fluke, which closely resembles *H. heterophyes* in size, form, life-cycle and pathogenesis, is very common in the Far East, and has also been reported from Spain, the Balkan States and Palestine. The snail host is *Semisulcospira libertina*. Man contracts the infection by eating infected raw or under-cooked fish. Various fish-eating birds and mammals, including the pelican, are reservoir hosts.

Echinostomum ilocanum (**Garrison's fluke**). This is another small fluke which occurs in India, China and the South East Asian islands, but only infects man in Java, Celebes and the Philippine Islands. The first intermediate host is a water-snail belonging to one of the three genera *Gyraulus*, *Hippeutis* or *Lymnaea*. The second intermediate host, in which the cercariae encyst, is also a fresh-water mollusc, usually *Pila* spp. in the Philippines or *Viviparus javanicus* in Java. Man acquires the infection by eating the infected second intermediate host raw or under-cooked. Dogs and field rats are reservoir hosts.

Troglotrema salmincola. This is a very small (0·04 by 1 mm) fluke which normally parasitises the mucous layers of the intestine in fish-eating mammals (dog, coyote, fox, raccoon, mink and lynx) on the Pacific Coast of North America and in Eastern Siberia. The first intermediate host in the United States is the snail *Galba silicula*, the second a salmonoid fish. The infection is acquired by eating raw or insufficiently cooked infected fish. Human infection is mild and relatively infrequent, but in animal hosts the fluke transmits a highly pathogenic virus which causes an acute febrile syndrome characterised by severe haemorrhagic enteritis, complete anorexia, uncontrollable vomiting and bloody dysentery, and generally terminating fatally.

A large number of trematode species infect the alimentary tract of various species of domestic animals. Some of the more important are shown in Table 3.

Hepatic Trematodes

The following trematode species infect the human liver:

Clonorchis sinensis (**Chinese** or **Oriental liver-fluke**). This is a medium-sized (7–20 mm) fluke which inhabits the bile-ducts of man in the Far East, principally in China, Formosa, Japan, Korea and Indo-China. The eggs pass out in the faeces and hatch if swallowed by the appropriate aquatic snail (species of *Parafossarulus*, *Bulinus* and *Alocinma*). The parasite passes through sporocyst and redia

TABLE 3

Parasite	Definitive hosts	Location in hosts	Intermediate hosts	Pathogenic effects	Comment
ECHINOSTOMATIDAE					
Echinostoma revolutum	Ducks, geese, fowls, partridges (man)	Rectum, caeca	Various species of aquatic snails	Enteritis	
Echinoparyphium paraulum	Ducks, pigeons, (man)	Small intestine	Unknown	Enteritis, diarrhoea, weakness	
E. recurvatum	Ducks, fowls, pigeons	Duodenum	1. Aquatic snails 2. Frogs and other species of snails	Enteritis, emaciation, anaemia and weakness	
Hypoderaeum conoideum	Ducks, geese, swans, fowls, pigeons	Ileum	1. Aquatic snails 2. Frogs and tadpoles	Enteritis, emaciation, anaemia, weakness	
Echinochasmus perfoliatus	Dogs, cats, foxes, pigs	Intestine	1. Aquatic snails 2. Freshwater fish	Enteritis	Europe, Asia
Euparyphium melis	Cats, foxes, mink, and other fur-bearers*	Small intestine	1. Water-snails 2. Tadpoles	Haemorrhagic enteritis in mink	
HETEROPHYIDAE					
Heterophyes heterophyes	Dogs, cats, foxes (man)		See above		
Metagonimus yokogawai	Dogs, cats, pigs (man)		See above		
Euryhelmis squamula	Foxes and other fur-bearers	Intestine	1. Unknown 2. Frogs	Fatal enteritis in mink	
E. monorchis	Mink	Intestine	1. Aquatic snails 2. Frogs	Enteritis	
Cryptocotyle lingua	Cats, dogs and fur-bearers. Fish-eating birds	Intestine	Unknown—probably fish (sea)	Enteritis	North Sea area

PLAGIORCHIDAE					
Prosthogonimus pellucidus and other species of this genus	Fowls, ducks	Posterior intestine (Bursa fabricii). Enter oviduct in laying birds	1. Snails 2. Dragonflies	Inflammation of oviduct, peritonitis	Most serious trematode parasite of poultry in Europe and America
Plagiorchis megalorchis	Turkeys	Posterior intestine (as *P. pellucidus*)	1. Aquatic snails 2. Midges	Inflammation of oviduct, peritonitis	
NOTOCOTYLIDAE					
Notocotylus attenuatus	Fowls, ducks, geese	Caeca, rectum	Water-snails		
Catatropis verrucosa	Fowls, ducks, geese	Caeca	Water-snails	Inflammation of caecal mucosa	
Cymbiforma indica	Sheep, goats, cattle	Duodenum, stomach, intestine	Unknown	Duodenitis	India
BRACHYLAEMIDAE					
Brachylaemus commutatus	Fowls, guinea fowls, pheasants, turkeys, pigeons	Caeca	Land snails?	Caecal inflammation	South Europe, North Africa, Indo-China
B. suis	Pigs	Small intestine	Land snails	Enteritis	North Africa
Skrjabinotrema ovis	Sheep	Ileum	Unknown	Enteritis, debility, diarrhoea	China
TROGLOTREMATIDAE					
Paragonimus spp.	Cats, pigs, dogs	As for *P. westermani* (see below)			
Troglotrema salmincola	Dogs, foxes and fur-bearers	Small intestine	1. Water-snails 2. Salmonoid fish	Enteritis—transmits fatal virus infection	China

* Fur-bearers are chiefly carnivorous mammals belonging to the families Canidae (silver, black and blue foxes) and Mustelidae (weasel, ermine, stoat, ferret, raccoon, marten, fisher, skunk, mink and otter) together with some rodents (squirrels, rabbits, beaver, musk-rat) and the marsupial opossum. Little investigation of the parasitic diseases affecting these animals has been made except in the case of those which are reared on fur-farms (foxes, mink).

TABLE 3 (continued)

Parasite	Definitive hosts	Location in hosts	Intermediate hosts	Pathogenic effects	Comment
PARAMPHISTOMATIDAE					
Paramphistomum cervi and related species	Sheep, goats, cattle	Rumen, reticulum	Aquatic snails	Mucosal inflammation	
Cotylophoron cotylophorum	Sheep, goats, cattle	Rumen, reticulum	Aquatic snails	Mucosal irritation, diarrhoea, anaemia, weakness	
Calicophoron sp., *Ceylonocotyle* sp., *Gastrothylax* spp., *Fischoederius* spp., *Carmyerius* spp.	Sheep, goats, cattle	Rumen	Unknown	Not usually serious but *Fischoederius* said to be fatal in cattle	Southern Asia, Far East
Gastrodiscus aegyptiacus	Horses, pigs	Small and large intestines	Aquatic snails	Not serious	
Gastrodiscoides hominis	Pigs (man)	See above			
STRIGEIDAE					
Apatemon gracilis	Pigeons, ducks	Intestine	1. Snails 2. Leeches	Not serious	
Parastrigea robusta	Ducks	Intestine	Unknown	Haemorrhagic enteritis—diarrhoea, anaemia	
Cotylurus cornutus	Pigeons, ducks	Small intestine	Aquatic snails	Haemorrhagic enteritis—diarrhoea	

generations in the tissues of the snail to reach the cercaria stage, which leaves the first intermediate host and penetrates beneath the scales of a fresh-water fish to encyst as a metacercaria in the superficial musculature. A great many species of fresh-water fish can serve as second intermediate host. When the fish is eaten by a suitable definitive host the metacercariae excyst in the duodenum and migrate up the bile-duct to the liver, there to develop into adults. Man acquires the infection by eating raw, pickled or inadequately cooked infected fish. Many fish-eating mammals act as reservoir hosts, including dog, fox, cat, pig, rat and various wild species. Heavy infections are characterised by cirrhotic thickening and fibrosis of the walls of the affected bile-ducts, necrosis and pressure atrophy of adjacent liver parenchyma, with resulting jaundice and systemic toxaemia. Symptoms include jaundice, diarrhoea, oedema and painful, progressive hepatomegaly.

Opisthorchis tenuicollis **(Cat liver-fluke).** This parasite closely resembles *C. sinensis* both morphologically and in its life-cycle, the principal differences lying in the testes, which are not branched. It is widely distributed in Europe and occurs also in many parts of Asia, but is rare in areas where *C. sinensis* is endemic. Human infection is most frequent in Prussia and Siberia. The first intermediate host is a species of the water-snail genus *Bulimus*. Almost any species of fresh-water fish may serve as second intermediate host. Infection is acquired by man in the same way as *C. sinensis* infection. The pathogenic effects of the two parasites are identical.

Fasciola hepatica **(Sheep liver-fluke).** This cosmopolitan species is primarily a parasite of sheep and goats, in which it causes the disease known as **liver-rot;** but human infections occur from time to time in most endemic areas. It is a large (2–3 by 1 cm), leaf-shaped fluke which lives in the bile-ducts of the host, causing similar pathogenic effects and symptoms to the two preceding species. Toxaemia, however, is usually more marked. Pharyngeal infection with young flukes **(halzoun)** may occur in man if infected liver is eaten raw; but this is rare. Liver-rot is a scourge in damp sheep-farming areas in many parts of the world, often causing the death of the hosts. Human infection, however, is rarely severe and still more rarely fatal. The life-cycle is similar to that of *C. sinensis* but involves only a single intermediate host, which is usually a water-snail belonging to the genus *Lymnaea* (*L. truncatula* in Great Britain). Two redial generations may occur. The cercariae encyst on wet grass or submerged vegetation, which is subsequently eaten by the definitive host. Man usually acquires the infection by consuming infested water-cress. Cattle and a number of other domestic and wild herbivores may also become infected.

Dicrocoelium dendriticum (**Lanceolate fluke**). This is a small (10 by 2 mm) lanceolate fluke of cosmopolitan distribution. It occurs

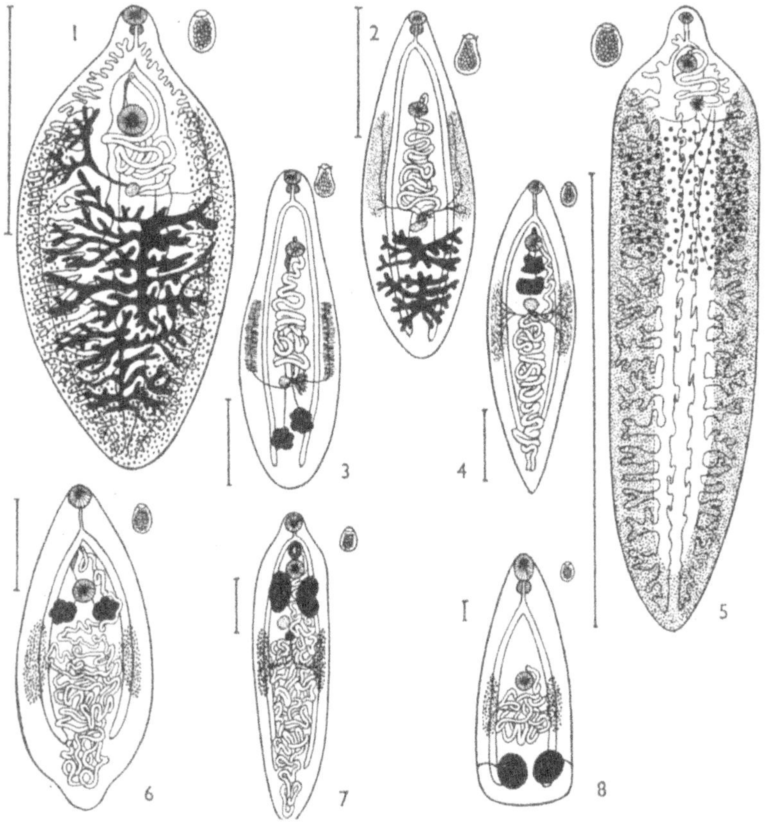

FIG. 8. Liver Flukes and their eggs

1 *Fasciola hepatica.*
2 *Opisthorchis tenuicollis.*
3 *Clonorchis sinensis.*
4 *Dicrocoelium dendriticum.*
5 *Fasciola gigantica.*
6 *Eurytrema pancreaticum.*
7 *Platynosomum concinnum.*
8 *Pseudomphistomum truncatum.*

principally in cattle, sheep and goats. Genuine human infections are rare, but spurious ones occur not infrequently. The life-cycle is peculiar in that the eggs, after leaving the definitive host in the faeces, hatch only if ingested by an appropriate species of land-snail, such as *Cionella lubrica*, in which the parasite passes through

TABLE 4

Parasite	Definitive hosts	Location in hosts	Intermediate hosts	Pathogenic effects	Comment
DICROCOELIDAE					
Dicrocoelium dendriticum	Sheep, goats, cattle, pigs, dogs, donkeys, rabbits	Liver and bile-ducts	See above		
Platynosomum concinnum	Cats	Liver and bile-ducts	Unknown	Inflammation of bile-ducts, hepatomegaly, loss of appetite, death	Malay States, British Guiana, Brazil
Eurytrema pancreaticum	Sheep, goats, cattle	Liver and bile-ducts	1. Land snails 2. *Unknown*	Inflammation and occlusion of infected ducts, poor condition	Eastern Asia, Brazil
OPISTHORCHIDAE					
Opisthorchis tenuicollis	Dogs, cats, foxes, pigs (man)	Bile-ducts and pancreatic duct	See above		
Clonorchis sinensis	Dogs, cats, pigs (man), fur-bearers	Bile-ducts	See above		
Pseudomphistomum truncatum	Dogs, cats, foxes	Liver and bile-ducts	1. Fresh-water snails 2. Fresh-water fish		Europe, India
FASCIOLIDAE					
Fasciola hepatica	Sheep, goats, cattle, etc.	See above		Digestive, disturbances, anaemia, emaciation, weakness, death	
F. gigantica	As *F. hepatica*				
Fascioloides magna	Cattle, horses, bison, yaks	Liver and bile-ducts	Fresh-water snails	Varies—severe in sheep	N. America, Europe

two sporocyst generations to reach the cercarial stage. The cercariae leave the snail during rainy weather in masses of mucus known as slime-balls, and must then be ingested by a second intermediate host, the common brown ant, *Formica fusca*. The definitive host becomes infected by accidentally swallowing infected brown ants. Pathogenesis, both in man and domestic animals, is less severe than in other forms of liver-fluke infection.

A number of trematode species infect the liver of domestic animals, as set forth in Table 4.

Pulmonary Trematodes

There is only one important trematode parasite of the human lung.

Paragonimus westermani (**Oriental lung-fluke**). This is a plump, fleshy, ovoid fluke of medium size (8–16 by 4–8 by 3–5 mm), having a spiny integument. It is common in man in many parts of the Far East, including China, Japan, Korea, Formosa and South-East Asia, occurring encapsulated in the lungs. The eggs are coughed up and either voided in the sputum or swallowed and discharged in the faeces. They hatch in water and the miracidium penetrates the first intermediate host, a water-snail belonging to the genus *Semisulcospira*, in which the sporocyst and two redial generations are passed. The cercariae escape and penetrate the second intermediate host, which is a fresh-water crab or crayfish. Man acquires the infection either by eating infected crabs or crayfish raw, salted or pickled, or by consuming other food contaminated with the parasite during the preparation of crab soup. There are many reservoir

TABLE 5

Parasite	Definitive hosts	Location in hosts	Intermediate hosts	Pathogenic effect	Comment
TROGLOTREMATIDAE					
Paragonimus westermani	Pigs, dogs, cats, goats, cattle fur-bearers	See above			
CYCLOCOELIDAE					
Typhlocoelum cymbium and other species of this genus	Ducks	Trachea, bronchi	Fresh-water snails	Dyspnoea and asphyxia	

hosts since the parasite is able to develop to maturity in almost any species of crab- or crayfish-eating mammal. Infection is accompanied by pulmonary inflammation and fibrosis with a resulting pneumonia-like syndrome and persistant cough.

Lung-fluke infections occurring in domestic animals are shown in Table 5.

Blood Trematodes

Three species of the trematode genus *Schistosoma* are important parasites of the human circulatory system in warm climates, namely:

S. haematobium (Africa and the Middle East, Madagascar and Mauritius).
S. mansoni (Africa and the Middle East, West Indies, South America).
S. japonicum (Far East especially China, Japan, Formosa, Celebes and the Philippines).

The adult worms of all three species live in the visceral veins, to which they are adapted by their long, narrow, shape (male 8–15 by 0·5–1 mm) (female 20 by 0·25 mm). The edges of the broader body of the male are curved ventrad to form a gynaecophoric groove in which the longer, narrower, threadlike female lies. The spined eggs are laid in the venules in the wall of either the urinary bladder (*S. haematobium*) or the intestine and rectum (*S. mansoni* and *S. japonicum*); and work their way through the tissues to escape in the urine or the faeces. They hatch in water and the miracidium penetrates an appropriate species of snail:

S. haematobium—water-snails belonging to the genus *Bulinus*;
S. mansoni—water-snails belonging to the genus *Biomphalaria* in Africa and the Middle East, and to the genera *Australorbis* and *Tropicorbis* in South America;
S. japonicum—amphibious snails belonging to the genus *Oncomelania*.[1]

Within the snail the parasite passes through two sporocyst generations, the second of which gives rise to the cercaria. The cercaria, after escaping from the snail, swims about actively and

[1] Eggs of *S. haematobium* are elongate-oval and carry a terminal spine; those of *S. mansoni* are also elongate-oval but carry a lateral spine; while those of *S. japonicum* are oval but less elongate and carry a lateral hook.

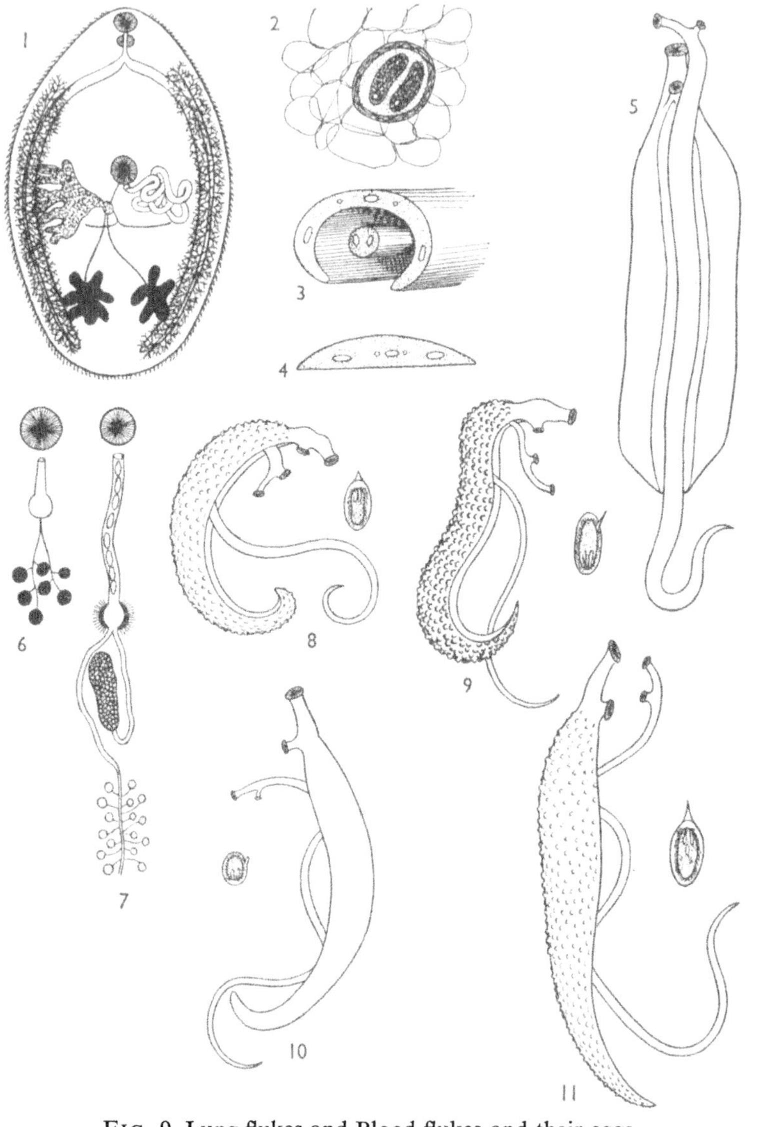

FIG. 9. Lung-flukes and Blood-flukes and their eggs

1 *Paragonimus westermani*—adult.
2 Section of lung showing two *P. westermani* enclosed in fibrous capsule filled with pus.
3 Diagrammatic solid section to show position of female blood-fluke in gynaecophoric groove of male.
4 Transverse section of male schistosome, opened out.
5 Ventral view of a pair of schistosomes, showing female lying in gynaecophoric groove of male.
6 Ventral sucker and reproductive organs of male schistosome (diagrammatic).

penetrates the skin of the definitive host, whence it is carried by the venous circulation to the heart and thence via the pulmonary circulation to the mesenteric vessels and liver, there to reach maturity.

S. japonicum occurs in a wide variety of mammalian species in addition to man, including dogs, cats, pigs, goats, horses, cattle and water-buffaloes, and a number of wild species; but reservoir hosts are of little importance in the cases of the other two species.

In *S. haematobium* infection the principal lesions occur in the wall of the urinary bladder. The tissues become heavily infiltrated with eggs, leading to haemorrhage, ulceration, fibrosis and eventually calcification. Common complications include blockage of the ureters and involvement of the genital system. Terminal haematuria is the most conspicuous early symptom, but tends to disappear as the disease progresses. Micturition becomes painful and difficult, and lower abdominal pain is a constant feature. In *S. mansoni* and *S. japonicum* infection similar lesions develop in the wall of the intestine, especially the caecum, colon and rectum. In heavy infections large numbers of eggs are carried back through the portal system to the liver, producing fibrotic lesions, periportal cirrhosis and hepatomegaly. Congestion and enlargement of the spleen follow. Pulmonary lesions and fever may also occur, both during the incubation period and later. Lesions and symptoms are more serious in *S. japonicum* infection than in Mansonian schistosomiasis, and the disease runs a more rapid course. Toxaemia, in particular, is more marked.

Schistosomiasis is one of the major tropical diseases of the world, affecting tens of millions of persons and ranking second in importance only to malaria.

Related forms affect domestic animals as shown in Table 6.

Skin Trematodes

In many parts of the world, including both temperate and tropical regions, an inflammatory condition of the skin, properly referred to as **schistosome dermatitis,** is caused by the attempted penetration of the cercariae of species of schistosomes normally parasitic as adults in birds or mammals other than man. Species of the genus *Trichobilharzia* are mainly involved. This form of itch is

---

7 Ventral sucker and reproductive organs of female schistosome (diagrammatic).
8 *Schistosoma haematobium*—male, female and egg.
9 *Schistosoma mansoni*—male, female and egg.
10 *Schistosoma japonicum*—male, female and egg.
11 *Schistosoma bovis*—male, female and egg.

TABLE 6

Parasite	Definitive hosts	Location in hosts	Intermediate hosts	Pathogenic effects†	Comments
Schistosoma japonicum	Dogs, cats, pigs, goats, horses, cattle		See above		
S. mattheei	Cattle, sheep, goats (man)	Visceral veins, especially mesenteric and portal	Fresh-water snails*	Lesions as in *S. japonicum*. Anaemia, fever, abdominal pain, anorexia, emaciation, death	Africa
S. bovis	Cattle, sheep, goats	,,	,,	,,	Africa, Middle East
S. leiperi	Cattle	,,	,,	,,	Kenya
S. rodhaini	Dogs, cats, rodents	,,	,,	,,	Africa
S. spindalis	Cattle, sheep, goats, dogs	,,	,,	,,	India, South-East Asia
S. indicum	Sheep, goats, cattle, camels, equines	,,	,,	,,	India
S. suis	Pigs, dogs	,,	,,	,,	India
Ornithobilharzia turkestanicum	Sheep, goats, cattle, cats, equines, camels	,,	,,	,,	Middle East, Central and Eastern Asia, Southern Europe
O. bomfordi	Zebu	,,	,,	,,	India
Schistosoma spindalis	Sheep, goats, cattle, dogs	Veins of the nasal mucosa	Fresh-water snails	Nasal granuloma	India
Bilharziella polonica	Ducks	Mesenteric and pelvic veins	,,	Slight	Europe, North America

* The species of fresh-water snails involved are members of the genera *Lymnaea*, *Planorbis*, *Indoplanorbis*, *Bulinus*, *Physopsis* and *Oncomelania*.

† Pathogenicity naturally varies with the severity of the infection and is generally less marked in large animals. Many cases are symptomless.

chiefly contracted by swimmers, agricultural labourers, sportsmen and collectors, bathers, fishermen, clam-diggers and others whose activities bring them frequently into contact with infested water. There are no systemic symptoms and the condition is self-terminating after a while.

Treatment and Prevention

The treatment of fluke diseases, both in man and animals, is still a matter of doubt and difficulty. Hexylresorcinol, piperazine, extract of male fern, tetrachlorethylene and carbon tetrachloride are used in the treatment of intestinal fluke infections. Trivalent antimonials such as intravenous sodium antimony tartrate and intramuscular fouadin, and a variety of oral drugs such as gentian violet, hexachlorethane, chloroquin, hexachlorophane, tetrachlorodifluoroethane, and intramuscular emetine hydrochloride are used against liver-fluke infections in animals, and the less toxic of these drugs are also used in human treatment. No really effective drug against lung-fluke infection in either man or animals has yet been found, but beneficial results are claimed for intramuscular emetine hydrochloride in conjunction with Prontosil soluble and for intravenous sodium antimony tartrate in cases of paragonimiasis westermani, and for sulphanilamide in animal infection with *Troglotrema salmincola*. Apomorphine administered within three hours of eating the infected fish is also stated to arrest *Troglotrema* infection in animals; and claims have been made for the use of immune serum. No treatment exists for lung-fluke infection in birds. Paramphistomes are also highly resistant to all known forms of treatment. In schistosomiasis the use of intravenous or intramuscular trivalent antimonials (sodium and potassium antimony tartrates, stibophen and trivalent sodium antimony gluconate) is still the treatment of choice, although the miracils are effective against certain forms of the disease when administered orally. Various substances have been used effectively as repellents against schistosome cercariae, e.g. dimethyl phthallate, dibutyl phthallate, copper oleate, benzyl benzoate and *NN* diethyl lauramide.

Prevention of trematode diseases involves:

(1) Elimination of the molluscan intermediate hosts (see section on Malacology).
(2) Mass treatment of all infected persons or animals so as to eliminate the sources of infection.

(3) Abstention from drinking unboiled or unfiltered water and from eating raw or insufficiently cooked vegetables, fish, meat or shellfish, or food prepared concurrently with such dishes, and the application of similar restrictions to animals, where these are the carriers of the infective stage.
(4) Prevention of promiscuous defaecation and the use of human faeces (night-soil) as fertiliser (unless previously treated with ammonium sulphate or otherwise sterilised).
(5) Sanitary disposal of human faeces.
(6) Organisation of animal care so that they are unable to eat infected second intermediate hosts and are kept away from marshy ground where certain types of infection may occur (especially schistosomiasis).
(7) Avoidance of contact with water infested with schistosome cercariae.

CESTOIDEA
(TAPEWORMS)

General

The Cestoidea are divided into two sub-classes known as the Cestodaria and the Eucestoda. The former have an undivided body and no scolex, whereas the latter have a scolex with organs of attachment, and a long, ribbon-like body consisting of many short sections termed proglottides. Each proglottide contains one or

---

FIG. 10. Life-cycle of Cestoda (generalised)

Upper figure—Pseudophyllidean Cycle.

1 Enlarged proglottides of adult worm.
2 Adult worm (develops in intestine of definitive host after ingestion of infected second intermediate host).
3 Egg (passes out in faeces and hatches in water).
4 Coracidium larva (free-swimming in water and is swallowed by first intermediate host).
5 Onchosphere (hexacanth) larva (liberated in gut of first intermediate host).
6 Procercoid larva (develops in body of first intermediate host).
7 Plerocercoid (sparganum) larva (develops in body of second intermediate host after ingestion of infected first intermediate host).

Lower figure—Cyclophyllidean Cycle.

1 Enlarged proglottides of adult worm.
2 Adult worm (develops in intestine of definitive host after ingestion of infected intermediate host).
3 Egg (passes out in faeces onto ground and does not hatch until ingested by intermediate host).
4 Onchosphere (hexacanth) larva (liberated in gut of intermediate host).
5 Cysticercus larva (develops in body of intermediate host).
N.B. invaginated scolex.
6 Cysticercus larva (starting to develop into adult worm in intestine of definitive host).

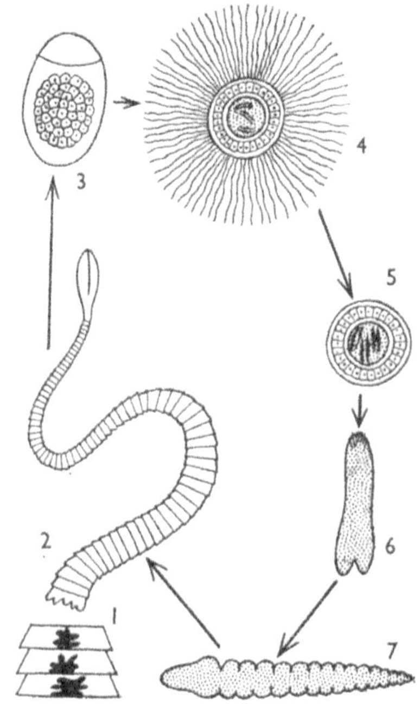
3
4
5
6
7
2
1

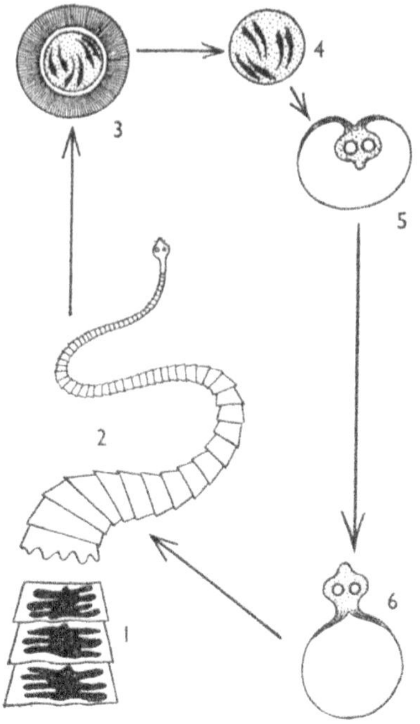
3
4
5
2
6
1

more complete sets of hermaphrodite reproductive organs. The forms of importance in human and veterinary medicine all belong to two of the nine orders into which the sub-class Eucestoda is divided, namely, the Pseudophyllidea and the Cyclophyllidea or Taenioidea. In the Pseudophyllidea the scolex is usually provided with two shallow, elongate, sucking-grooves **(bothria)**; whereas in Cyclophyllidea, the scolex is generally provided with four muscular, cup-like suckers **(acetabula)** and a mobile, muscular rostellum armed with hooks. The life-cycles also differ.

An adult pseudophyllidean tapeworm lives in the small intestine of the vertebrate definitive host and gives rise to eggs which escape in the faeces and hatch in water. A free-swimming, ciliated larva emerges which is known as a **coracidium.** If this is ingested by the first intermediate host which is a crustacean, the ciliated coat is shed and a six-hooked **onchosphere** or **hexacanth larva** emerges and burrows into the host tissues, where it develops into an elongate, muscular **procercoid larva.** No further development takes place unless the infected crustacean is swallowed by a suitable second intermediate host, which is a fresh-water fish. In this case the procercoid larva penetrates the intestinal wall as soon as it is freed by digestion of the crustacean, and develops in the tissues or body cavity of the fish into a **plerocercoid** or **sparganum larva.** If the infected fish is eaten by an appropriate definitive host the plerocercoid larva in its turn is liberated by digestion of the fish tissues and proceeds to attach itself to the intestinal wall, where it buds off a chain of proglottides.

An adult cyclophyllidean tapeworm also lives in the small intestine of the vertebrate definitive host and produces eggs which escape in the faeces, either singly or by the discharge of the complete proglottide containing them. The eggs hatch only after ingestion by the intermediate host, liberating an **onchosphere larva** which bores through the intestinal wall into the tissues and there develops into a vesicular stage which may be either a **cysticercoid** or a **cysticercus (bladder-worm).** This stage is distinguished by possessing a scolex which is normally orientated in a cysticercoid but introverted in a cysticercus. When the infected intermediate host is eaten by the definitive host, the larva is liberated by the digestion of the surrounding tissues, the scolex attaches itself to the gut wall and begins to bud off proglottides.

Adult Tapeworms in Man and Domestic Animals

There are six species of tapeworms which are common and important parasites of the human alimentary tract in the adult stage:

Diphyllobothrium latum **(the broad fish tapeworm).** This is a large (3–10 metres) pseudophyllidean tapeworm having a small (1–3 mm) ovoid scolex provided with two bothria and upwards of 3000 short, broad proglottides. It occurs mainly in the cooler parts of the northern hemisphere where food fish of fresh waters are often infected. The first intermediate host is a species of water-flea (*Cyclops* or *Diaptomus*). Many species of fresh-water fish including pike, salmon, trout, perch, burbot and pickerel, can act as second intermediate hosts. Many species of fish-eating mammals act as reservoir definitive hosts. Man acquires the infection by eating raw or under-cooked infected fish. The pathogenic effects of this parasite include intestinal catarrh, toxaemic symptoms and, in some cases, pernicious anaemia.

Taenia saginata **(the beef tapeworm).** This is a large (4–25 metres) cyclophyllidean tapeworm having a small (1–2 mm) pyriform scolex provided with four acetabula but lacking a rostellum and hooks. There may be 2000 or more almost square proglottides (9–12 mm), which become detached and leave the anus by their own movements. It is cosmopolitan in distribution. Cattle are the usual intermediate hosts. There are no known reservoir hosts. Man acquires the infection by eating raw or under-cooked beef infected with the bladder-worm stage (*Cysticercus bovis*). The infection is often symptomless, but abdominal discomfort, hunger pains, anorexia and diarrhoea or constipation may occur.

Taenia solium **(the pork tapeworm).** This species is closely related to the beef tapeworm but is somewhat smaller (2–7 metres), has a scolex provided with a rostellum carrying a double row of 22 to 32 hooklets in addition to the four acetabula, and generally has less than 1000 proglottides. It is cosmopolitan in distribution. Pigs are the usual intermediate hosts. Man acquires the infection by eating raw or under-cooked pork or pork products infected with the bladder-worm stage (*Cysticercus cellulosae*).

Hymenolepis nana **(the dwarf tapeworm).** This is a small (7–40 mm) cyclophyllidean tapeworm of cosmopolitan distribution having a minute (0·3 mm) globular scolex provided with four suckers and an invaginable rostellum carrying a single ring of 20 to

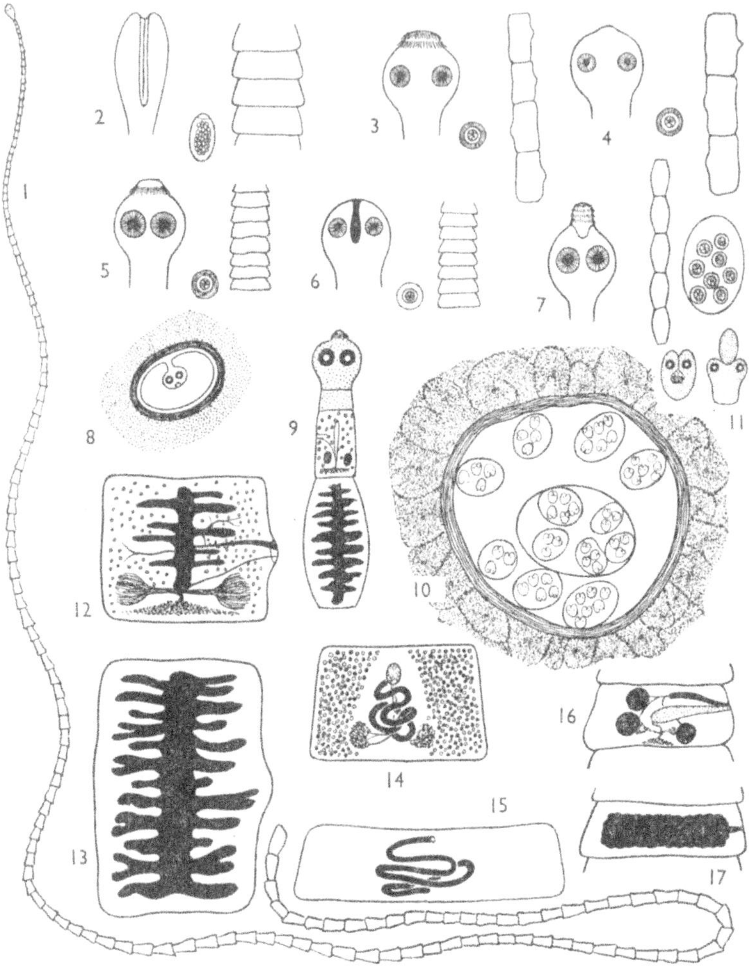

FIG. 11. Common Cestode Parasites of Man

1 Complete specimen of taenioid tapeworm showing scolex and strobila.
2 Scolex, egg and proglottides of *Diphyllobothrium latum.*
3 Scolex, egg and proglottides of *Taenia solium.*
4 Scolex, egg and proglottides of *Taenia saginata.*
5 Scolex, egg and proglottides of *Hymenolepis nana.*
6 Scolex, egg and proglottides of *Hymenolepis diminuta.*
7 Scolex, egg-sac and proglottides of *Dipylidium caninum.*
8 *Cysticercus cellulosae* encysted in human brain.
9 *Echinococcus granulosus* complete adult.
10 Hydatid cyst with brood capsules and scolices and an endogenous daughter cyst, embedded in human liver.
11 Hydatid scolices inverted (left) and everted (right).
12 Mature proglottide of *Taenia solium*, showing reproductive organs.
13 Gravid proglottide of *Taenia solium*, showing distended uterus and branches.

30 hooklets. There are upwards of 200 proglottides which are broader than long. No intermediate host is required, the bladderworm developing within the tissues of the intestinal villi of the definitive host. Rats, mice and hamsters act as reservoir hosts. Man acquires the infection by swallowing the eggs inadvertently in contaminated water or food or through oral contact with unclean hands. Light infections are symptomless but heavy infections are often associated with toxaemic symptoms such as abdominal pain, diarrhoea, headache and insomnia. The infection is commonest in children and certain types of institutional groups.

Hymenolepis diminuta (**the rat tapeworm**). This is a cosmopolitan parasite of rats and mice, closely related to the foregoing species, which not infrequently infects man. It is normally somewhat larger than *H. nana*; the scolex lacks rostellar hooks; and an intermediate host is necessary, which may be any one of a large number of meal- and grain-infesting insects or an insect directly associated with the rodent host. Cockroaches, rat-fleas and grain beetles are most often infected. Man, an accidental host, acquires the infection by accidentally ingesting infected insects when eating uncooked cereal foods. Symptoms are similar to those produced by *H. nana*.

Dipylidium caninum (**the common dog tapeworm**). This is a cosmopolitan parasite of cats and dogs which commonly infects children in certain parts of the world. It is a medium-sized (10–70 cm) tapeworm with a small (0·35 mm) rhomboidal scolex provided with four suckers and a retractile rostellum bearing 30 to 150 hooklets arranged in from one to seven rings. The elliptical proglottides, 60 to 175 in number, usually become detached when ripe and migrate out of the anus. Dog and cat-fleas (*Ctenocephalides canis* and *C. felis*), the human flea (*Pulex irritans*) and the dog louse (*Trichodectes canis*) act as intermediate hosts, becoming infected as larvae. Man acquires the infection by accidental ingestion of infected fleas or lice during contact with cats and dogs. The infection is generally symptomless, but a syndrome resembling that due to *H. nana* may occur.

A large number of adult tapeworms infect domestic animals. The important ones are shown in Table 7.

---

14 Mature proglottide of *Diphyllobothrium latum*, showing reproductive organs.
15 Gravid proglottide of *Diphyllobothrium latum*, showing uterine coils.
16 Mature proglottide of *Hymenolepis nana*, showing reproductive organs.
17 Gravid proglottide of *Hymenolepis nana*, showing distended uterus.

TABLE 7

Parasite	Definitive hosts	Intermediate hosts	Remarks
MESOCESTOIDIDAE			
Mesocestoides lineatus	Dogs, cats, fur-bearers	1. Coprophagous insect? 2. Vertebrate?	
ANOPLOCEPHALIDAE			
Anoplocephala spp.	Equines	Oribatid mites	
Paranoplocephala mamillana	Equines	Oribatid mites	
Moniezia spp.	Sheep, goats, cattle	Oribatid mites	
Cittotaenia spp.	Rabbits	Oribatid mites	
Avitellina spp.	Sheep, goats, cattle	Oribitad mites	Africa, Italy, India
Stilesia hepatica	Sheep, goats, cattle	Oribatid mites	Parasites creep into the bile-ducts, yet are almost non-pathogenic. Africa
Thysanosoma actinioides	Sheep, goats, cattle	Oribatid mites	Fringed tapeworm. U.S.A.
Helictometra giardi	Sheep, goats, cattle	Oribatid mites	Europe, Africa, America
DAVAINEIDAE			
Davainea proglottina	Fowls, pigeons, etc.	Slugs	
Raillietina proglottina	Fowls, guinea-fowls, pea-hens, pigeons	House-flies, ants	
R. echinobothrida	Fowls	Ants	
R. cesticillus	Fowls, turkeys, guinea-fowls	House-flies, beetles	
Cotugnia spp.	Fowls, ducks	Unknown	Fowl in Europe, Africa, Asia, duck in Burma, India
Houttuynia struthionis	Ostriches	Unknown	
DILEPIDIDAE			
Amoebotaenia sphenoides	Fowls	Earthworms	
Choanotaenia infundibulum	Fowls, turkeys	House-flies, beetles	
Dipylidium caninum	Cats, dogs (man)		See above
Joyeuxiella spp.	Cats	1. Dung beetles 2. Lizards and other reptiles	
Diplopylidium spp.			

TABLE 7 (continued)

Parasite	Definitive hosts	Intermediate hosts	Remarks
HYMENOLEPIDIDAE			
Hymenolepis nana	Rats, mice		See above
H. diminuta	(man)		
H. lanceolata *H. carioca* and many other species of this genus	Fowls, ducks, geese and other domestic birds	Arthropods—fresh-water crustacea (e.g. *Cyclops*) if definitive host is a water-bird; grain-beetles, etc. (e.g. *Aphodius*) if definitive host is a land-bird	
Fimbriaria fasciolaris	Fowls, ducks, geese	Copepods (e.g. *Cyclops* and *Diaptomus*)	
TAENIIDAE			
Taenia solium	Man	Pigs (*Cysticercus cellulosae*). See above	
T. saginata	Man	Cattle (*Cysticercus bovis*). See above	
T. hydatigena (*T. marginata*)	Dogs, fur-bearers	Sheep, goats, cattle, pigs, hamsters, etc. (*Cysticercus tenuicollis* in liver, peritoneal cavity and mesenteries)	
T. pisiformis (*T. serrata*)	Dogs, fur-bearers	Rabbits and hares. (*Cysticercus pisiformis* in liver, peritoneal cavity and mesenteries)	
T. ovis	Dogs, fur-bearers	Sheep, goats. (*Cysticercus ovis* under the epicardium and the pleura of the diaphragm, in muscles, etc.)	
T. taeniaeformis (*T. crassicollis*)	Cats, fur-bearers	Rats, mice, rabbits, squirrels, etc. (*Cysticercus fasciolaris* in the liver)	
T. krabbei	Dogs	Reindeer (*Cysticercus tarandi* in the muscles)	
Multiceps multiceps	Dogs, fur-bearers	Sheep, goats, cattle, horses (*Coenurus cerebralis* in the brain and spinal cord, causing syndrome known as 'the staggers')	
M. serialis	Dogs, fur-bearers	Rabbits, hares, coypu rats, squirrels (*Coenurus serialis* in intermuscular tissue)	
Echinococcus granulosus	Dogs, cats, fur-bearers	Man and all domestic animals (Hydatid cyst). (See below.)	
E. multilocularis	Dogs, cats, fur-bearers	Field mice, voles, shrews and ground squirrels. (Multilocular or alveolar hydatid cyst.) (See below.)	

Larval Tapeworms in Man and Domestic Animals

Five kinds of tapeworms occur as larvae in man.

Sparganum spp. These are the plerocercoid larvae of various species of the genus *Diphyllobothrium* parasitic in dogs, cats and related wild forms. They normally occur in the subcutaneous connective tissue and between the muscles, causing oedematous and painful lesions; but any tissue except bone may be invaded. In some cases proliferation of the parasite within the host tissues occurs. Man acquires the infection either by ingestion of infected *Cyclops* (first intermediate host) or by contact with infected flesh of second intermediate hosts (frogs, pigs, etc.).

Hymenolepis nana. As already noted, the larvae of this species normally develop in the intestinal villi of the definitive host.

Cysticercus cellulosae. This form is the larval stage of *Taenia solium.* It occurs not uncommonly in man, infecting any organ or tissue and producing fibrotic lesions the effects of which vary according to their locations. The most dangerous form of the disease is cerebral infection, which leads to serious mental symptoms if the larvae die. Man acquires the infection by ingestion of *T. solium* eggs in contaminated food or water; or auto-infection may occur, in persons infected with the adult worm, by anus-to-mouth transfer of the eggs on dirty fingers, or by the movement of eggs or gravid proglottides back into the stomach by reverse peristalsis.

Echinococcus granulosus **(the dwarf dog tapeworm).** The adult of this species is a small (5–8 mm), cosmopolitan, cyclophyllidean tapeworm occurring in dogs. The scolex bears four suckers and a rostellum with 30 to 50 hooklets in two rings. There are only three proglottides. The larval stage normally occurs in sheep and other herbivores, but man is commonly infected in sheep-raising areas. The bladder-worm, known as a **hydatid cyst,** continues to develop slowly for many years, eventually reaching a very large size if its location in the body allows it to do so. Hollow brood capsules are produced within the cyst by a process of internal budding from the lining germinal membrane; and within each of these a number of scolices develop. Pressure on the mother cyst may lead to the formation of internal daughter and grand-daughter cysts in the same way, each of which develops brood capsules of its own. Rupture of brood capsules and daughter cysts may take place in older cysts, liberating the scolices, which form a granular deposit at the bottom of the mother cyst known as hydatid sand. Man acquires the infection by ingesting eggs from infected dogs through fondling or too intimate contact. Any type of tissue can be invaded, includ-

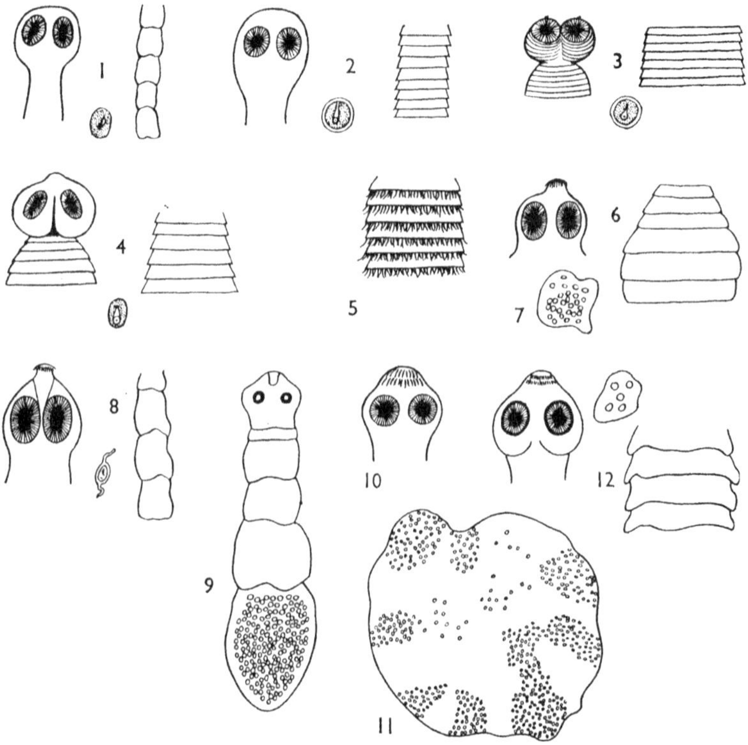

FIG. 12. Some Tapeworms of Domestic Animals

1 *Mesocestoides lineatus*—scolex, egg and proglottides.
2 *Moniezia expansa*—scolex, egg and proglottides.
3 *Anoplocephala magna*—scolex, egg and proglottides.
4 *Paranoplocephala mamillana*—scolex, egg and proglottides.
5 *Thysanosoma actinioides*—proglottides.
6 *Amoebotaenia sphenoides*—scolex and proglottides.
7 —egg-pouch with eggs.
8 *Choanotaenia infundibulum*—scolex, egg and proglottides.
9 *Davainea proglottina*—entire worm with gravid last proglottide full of eggs.
10 *Multiceps multiceps*—scolex.
11 *Coenurus cerebralis*—larval phase of *Multiceps multiceps* showing patches of scoleces on inside of bladder.
12 *Raillietina echinobothrida*—scolex, egg-pouch and proglottides.

ing bone. The pathological effects and symptoms depend upon the size and location of the cyst. They may be very serious in the case of large cysts in vital organs. Some 70 per cent of all cysts in man occur in the liver, about 20 per cent in the lungs, and the remainder in the kidney, spleen, abdominal cavity, brain, bones, subcutaneous tissues, muscles and heart. If a primary cyst ruptures, scolices and fragments of the germinal epithelium lining the cyst become disseminated through the body and may give rise to secondary cysts in other sites.

Echinococcus multilocularis. This form is closely related to the preceding species but the definitive hosts are wild foxes and the normal intermediate hosts field-mice and other small rodents. The larval stage, known as a multilocular or alveolar hydatid cyst, is an irregular spongy mass of small vesicles containing scolices and filled with a jelly-like matrix instead of fluid. It is neoplastic in nature, penetrating the tissues in a root-like manner and giving rise to metastases which are carried to other parts of the body in the blood or lymph, there to give rise to new cysts. Sporadic human cases are not uncommon.

Larval tapeworms infecting domestic animals are of relatively minor importance so far as veterinary medicine is concerned, but are in many cases a source of infection to man or to other domestic animals and are therefore of human and veterinary public health interest. The more important ones are listed in Table 7 above.

Treatment and Prevention

Human infection with adult tapeworms is usually treated with one of the following drugs, after twenty-four hours on a fluid diet to ensure adequate contact between drug and parasite:

Male Fern Extract
Kamala
Carbon tetrachloride
Hexylresorcinol by duodenal intubation
Stannoxyl
Mepacrine (Atebrine)
Acranil
Pelletierine
Tetrachlorethylene
Amadiaquine
Dithiazanine
2, 2′-dihydroxy-5, 5′-dichlorodiphenylmethane (Antiphen)

The drug of choice differs according to the nature and severity of the infection. Pre- and post-treatment purgation with a saline purgative increases efficacy by removing the mucus which might protect the parasites and ensuring their rapid evacuation before they can recover from the effects of the drug. In animal infections the same drugs are used and also:

Arecoline hydrobromide
Areca nut
Tin compounds, such as dibutyl tin dilaurate
Hexachlorophene
Nicotine and copper sulphate
Arsenates of lead, calcium, copper, cobalt and ferric iron
Various proprietary compounds such as Neguvon, Dichlorophen, Diphenthane 70 and Nemural).

The last-named group of drugs, together with the arsenates and the nicotine-copper sulphate mixture are the most effective against moniezіasis, while hexachlorophane, kamala, dibutyl tin dilaurate and carbon tetrachloride are the treatments of choice against tapeworm infections in poultry. Many cestodifugal or cestodicidal drugs are irritating to the gastric mucosa and are therefore administered in gelatine capsules. Human hydatid infection can only effectively be treated by surgery, although desensitisation is sometimes attempted.

Prevention of tapeworm infections involves avoiding consumption of infected intermediate hosts especially in the form of raw or under-cooked fish or meat by man, and prevention of this in the case of animals; sanitary disposal of faeces; and the maintenance of animal pens, stables and byres in a clean and hygienic condition. Pork can be sterilised against *Cysticercus cellulosae* by cooking, irradiation or sufficiently long deep freezing. Anti-rodent campaigns; care to avoid contamination of grain, rice, cereals, dried fruit and other stored food products with rodent excreta or the infestation of these materials with insects; campaigns against such intermediate hosts as cockroaches, fleas and grain insects; disinfestation of cats and dogs; and abstention from contact with pets; are all useful measures against infection with dog and rodent tapeworms and with larval stages. Strict de-worming of sheep-dogs and prevention of consumption of uncooked sheep offal by them is essential in the prevention of hydatid infection.

ACANTHOCEPHALA (THORNY-HEADED WORMS)

The **thorny-headed worms** include only two species that occur in the intestine of man.

Macracanthorhynchus hirudinaceus. This is a large (female 20–65 by 1 cm; male 5–10 by 0·5 cm), cosmopolitan form normally para-

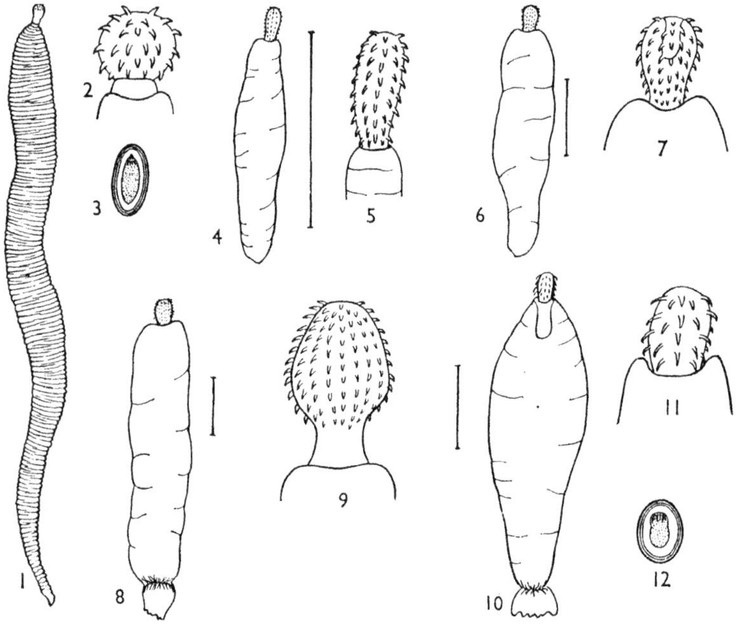

FIG. 13. Acanthocephalan Parasites of Man and Domestic Animals

1 *Macracanthorhynchus hirudinaceus*—adult female worm.
2 —evaginated proboscis.
3 —egg.
4 *Moniliformis moniliformis*—adult female worm.
5 —evaginated proboscis.
6 *Polymorphus boschadis*—adult female worm.
7 —evaginated proboscis.
8 *Filicollis anatis*—adult male worm.
9 —evaginated proboscis.
10 *Oncicola canis*—adult male worm.
11 —evaginated proboscis.
12 —egg.

sitic in pigs. Various species of dung-beetles (Scarabaeidae) serve as intermediate hosts. Human infection is rare.

Moniliformis moniliformis. This is another large (female 10–30 cm: male 4–13 cm) form of cosmopolitan distribution. The normal definitive host is the rat. Various species of beetles and cockroaches serve as intermediate hosts.

Man acquires both these infections by accidental ingestion of the infected intermediate host. The parasites cause ulceration and inflammation of the gut wall resulting in gastro-intestinal pain and diarrhoea.

Several species infect the intestinal tract of domestic animals (Table 8).

TABLE 8

Parasite	Definitive hosts	Intermediate hosts	Pathogenic effects
Macracanthorhynchus hirudinaceus	Pigs (man)	Dung-beetles (Scarabaeidae)	Slow growth, emaciation, perforation of gut and resulting peritonitis which may be fatal
Polymorphus boschadis	Ducks, swans, fowls, geese	Fresh-water shrimp (*Gammarus*) and perhaps crayfish	Anaemia, emaciation, cachexia, death
Filicollis anatis	Ducks, geese, swans	Fresh-water louse (*Asellus*)	Anaemia, emaciation, cachexia, death
Oncicola canis	Dogs (U.S.A.)	Unknown, perhaps armadillo?	Rabiform symptoms

Acanthocephalan infection in man is so rare that no real knowledge of effective treatment exists, but nicotine sulphate and carbon disulphide are said to have a beneficial effect in animal infections. Prevention clearly involves avoidance of ingestion of infected intermediate hosts.

NEMATODA

(ROUND-WORMS)

This is a very large class which is subdivided into 21 sub-orders, of which seven contain free-living species only, one contains plant-parasitic species and the remainder contain forms which are facultative or obligate parasites of animals.

The nematode life-cycle involves four juvenile stages separated by moults (see p. 72).

Any or all of the juvenile stages of the forms parasitic as adults in animals may be free-living or parasitic; and such great diversity consequently occurs in the life-cycle that lack of space forbids any general treatment of the subject here. It may be noted, however, that a juvenile is always present in the egg before hatching, which occurs at different stages of development in different species of nematodes.

First-stage juvenile
↓ first moult
Second-stage juvenile
↓ second moult
Third-stage juvenile (pre-adolescent stage)
↓ third moult
Fourth-stage juvenile (adolescent stage)
↓ fourth moult
Adult

Tylenchoidea

The members of this order are small nematodes parasitic on plants. Many species are crop parasites of great economic importance. The study of these forms has developed into a specialised branch of helminthology often referred to as nematology or phytonematology. Occasionally eggs of members of this group are found in human faeces as a result of consuming infected plants, and may be erroneously reported as human parasites (e.g. *Heterodera*). Consideration of the plant-parasitic eelworms is outside the scope of this work.

Rhabdiasoidea

A single species of this order is parasitic in man.

Strongyloides stercoralis. This is a cosmopolitan form which is more abundant in tropical and sub-tropical than in temperate climates because the free-living stages are favoured by warmth. Two distinct types of adult occur, namely, a free-living type and a parasitic type, differing somewhat in the details of their anatomy. The male of both types is a minute, fusiform worm, rarely exceeding 1 mm in length, whereas the free-living female, which is also fusiform, may be 10 mm long or more, and the slender filiform parasitic female 20–22 mm. The parasitic forms occur in the small intestine, where the female burrows into the mucosa after fertilisation and lays eggs which hatch *in situ*, the resulting juveniles escaping into the intestinal lumen and passing out in the faeces. In the stale faeces or soil they develop into free-living adults which mate and lay eggs in their turn. When the resulting juveniles reach the infective (filariform) stage they must penetrate the skin of the definitive host if the life-cycle is to continue. Thence they migrate through the venous circulation to the right heart and the lungs, where they escape from the capillaries into the air-sacs, ascend the respiratory tree to the pharynx and descend through the oesophagus and stomach to the intestine, where they become sexually mature adults. If external conditions are favourable the free-living phase tends to predominate and several free-living generations may succeed each other before reverting to the parasitic phase. Two forms of internal re-infection may also occur, in which a number of parasitic generations may succeed each other without the intervention of a free-living phase: in one, juvenile offspring of the parasitic adults may invade the intestinal mucosa, carry out a lung migration and return to the intestine to achieve maturity **(hyperinfection)**; while in the other, juveniles in the faeces may penetrate the peri-anal skin, thence to migrate through the lungs and respiratory tree in the usual way **(auto-infection).** Man acquires the infection by walking barefoot on contaminated soil or (more rarely) by accidental ingestion of infective juveniles. A pruritic skin lesion may be produced by the invading juveniles; such pulmonary symptoms as cough, bronchitis and pulmonitis are produced by juveniles migrating through the lungs; while adult worms in the intestine, if numerous, give rise to considerable mucosal inflammation with resulting diarrhoea, abdominal pain and generalised toxaemic symptoms. There are no reservoir hosts. Although a physiologically distinct race of *S. strongyloides* occurs in dogs, it is not transmissible to man.

Related species occur in a number of domestic animals:

S. papillosus in sheep, goats, cattle, rabbits and fur-bearers (highly pathogenic in mink),
S. westeri in equines and pigs,
S. cati in cats,
S. ransomi in pigs,
S. suis in pigs,
S. avium in small intestine and caeca of fowls and turkeys.

Severe infections with these various species cause enteritis, diarrhoea, weakness and, in young animals, stunting. Mild and moderate infections are usually symptomless.

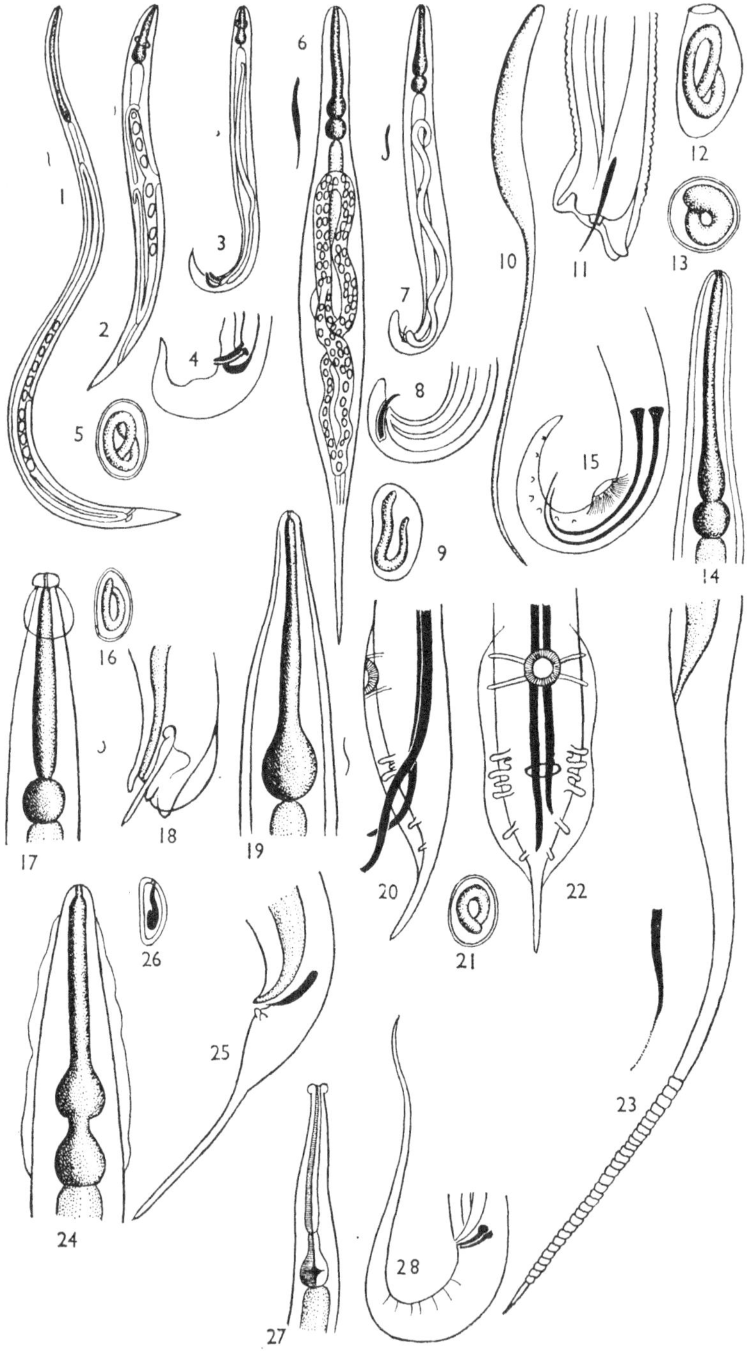

1
2
3
4
5
6
7
8
9
10
11
12
13
14
15
16
17
18
19
20
21
22
23
24
25
26
27
28

Until relatively recently the most effective drugs against *Strongyloides stercoralis* infection in man were gentian violet, preferably administered in solution by duodenal intubation, and diethylcarbamazine; but the discovery of dithiazanine has provided an effective weapon against this parasite. In animals phenothiazine has some effect provided that formulations with very fine particle size are employed; and organophosphorus compounds, tetrachlorethylene and hexylresorcinol are also used. Prevention in man is clearly a matter of sanitary disposal of faeces, and of not walking barefoot on ground that may be infested with infective juveniles. Sanitation and clean conditions in fowl-houses, byres, piggeries and stables are obviously the essential preventive measures in animal infections.

Oxyuroidea

A single species of this order is parasitic in man.

Enterobius vermicularis (**human pinworm** or **threadworm**). This is a cosmopolitan form which infects children more commonly than adults and is more frequent in cold climates than in warm ones. The adults, which inhabit the caecum, appendix and colon, are

---

FIG. 14. Rhabditoid and Oxyuroid Parasites

1 *Strongyloides stercoralis*—parasitic female.
2 —free-living female.
3 —free-living male.
4 —posterior extremity of free-living male, showing spicules (side view).
5 —egg.
6 *Enterobius vermicularis*—adult female.
7 —adult male.
8 —posterior extremity of male, showing spicule (side view).
9 —egg.
10 *Oxyuris equi*—adult female.
11 —posterior extremity of male, showing spicule (side view).
12 —egg.
13 *Subulura brumpti*—egg.
14 —anterior extremity of adult worm.
15 —posterior extremity of adult male, showing spicules (side view).
16 *Skrjabinema ovis*—egg.
17 —anterior extremity of adult worm.
18 —posterior extremity of adult male, showing spicule (side view).
19 *Heterakis gallinae*—anterior extremity of adult worm.
20 —posterior extremity of adult male, showing spicules, papillae and caudal alae (side view).
21 —egg.
22 —posterior extremity of adult male, showing spicules, papillae and caudal alae (ventral view).
23 *Passalurus ambiguus*—posterior extremity of adult female.
24 —anterior extremity of adult worm.
25 —posterior extremity of adult male, showing spicule (side view).
26 —egg.
27 *Probstmayria vivipara*—anterior extremity of adult worm.
28 —posterior extremity of adult male, showing spicules (side view).

small (2–13 by 0·1–0·5 mm) fusiform worms. The male is conspicuously smaller than the female. After fertilisation the gravid female migrates through the colon and rectum during the late evening or early night and, emerging through the anus, deposits her eggs on the peri-anal skin, whence they are subsequently dislodged by the movements of the host or by scratching. If they are then swallowed by a human being they hatch in the duodenum and the liberated juveniles pass slowly down the small intestine, completing their development on the way, so that they are mature by the time they reach the caecum. Man acquires the infection in one of the five following ways:

(*a*) Direct anus-to-mouth transmission by fingers contaminated by scratching the infected peri-anal skin **(re-infection).**
(*b*) Direct anus-to-mouth transmission by drawing soiled night clothes over the head **(re-infection).**
(*c*) Indirect anus-to-mouth transmission by transference of eggs from contaminated fingers to food, eating and drinking vessels and cigarettes **(re-infection and new infections).**
(*d*) Inhalation and swallowing of air-borne eggs in dust **(new infections).**
(*e*) Hatching of eggs on the peri-anal skin or anal mucosa and migration of the resulting juveniles back through the anus and up into the bowel **(retrofection).**

There are no important reservoir hosts. Only 5 per cent of infected children normally show symptoms, which are related more to the personality of the subject than to the heaviness of the infection, nervous children being more troubled than calm ones. Vague gastro-intestinal disturbances, anal irritation and irritable tiredness due to the resulting loss of sleep are the principal effects. Anal lesions may result from scratching and be made worse by secondary infection. Allegedly associated nervous symptoms must be discarded as not proven, since investigation has shown them to be as frequent in groups of uninfected children as in infected ones. Occasionally threadworms block the appendiceal lumen and appendicitis may then result.

A number of species of threadworms infect domestic animals, but none of them are seriously pathogenic:

Oxyuris equi in the large intestine of equines.
Passalurus ambiguus in the caecum and colon of rabbits and hares.
Skrjabinema spp. in the caecum of sheep and goats.

Probstmayria vivipara in the colon of equines gives birth to living offspring which grow to maturity without leaving the host intestine. This is the only known example of multiplication of a nematode within the host body. Very heavy infections result, but the parasite is nevertheless apparently not pathogenic.

Heterakis gallinae in the caeca of fowls, turkeys, ducks, geese and other birds. Diarrhoea and loss of condition may accompany this infection; but the parasite is more important as a vector of the protozoan *Histomonas meleagridis*, the cause of blackhead disease.

Subulura brumpti in the caeca of fowls, turkeys, guinea-fowls and other birds in Africa, South America and Spain. An insect intermediate host is involved, usually a beetle, earwig or cockroach.

This is another form of nematode infection which until recent times was refractory to all known forms of treatment. The discovery of the efficacy of the piperazine salts, however, opened up a new era, free as they are from noxious side-effects. Dithiazanine is also effective against oxyuriasis in man and animals; and certain cyanine dyes, notably pyrrovinyquinium pamoate (marketed as Povan), have now been added to the list of non-toxic oxyuricides.

Prevention in man involves extreme cleanliness, both personal and general; the liberal use of soap and water; frequent changes of under-clothes, night-clothes and bed-linen; swabbing of floors, shelves and ledges with antiseptic solutions; and avoidance of all anus-to-mouth contacts of any kind. In animals only *Heterakis gallinae* is of any serious pathogenic importance; and this infection must be combated by keeping poultry in the most hygienic conditions possible.

Ascaroidea

Only one species is regularly parasitic in man.

Ascaris lumbricoides. This cosmopolitan species, the commonest helminth parasite of man, is more frequent in warm than in cold climates and, like *Entamoeba histolytica*, shows high endemicity where standards of sanitation and personal hygiene are low. The adults are large (15–35 cm by 2–6 mm), fusiform worms, which lie free in the lumen of the small intestine, although they may attach themselves to the mucosa temporarily by means of their lips. The female is larger than the male. The thick-walled resistant eggs pass out in the faeces and must remain for several weeks in the soil

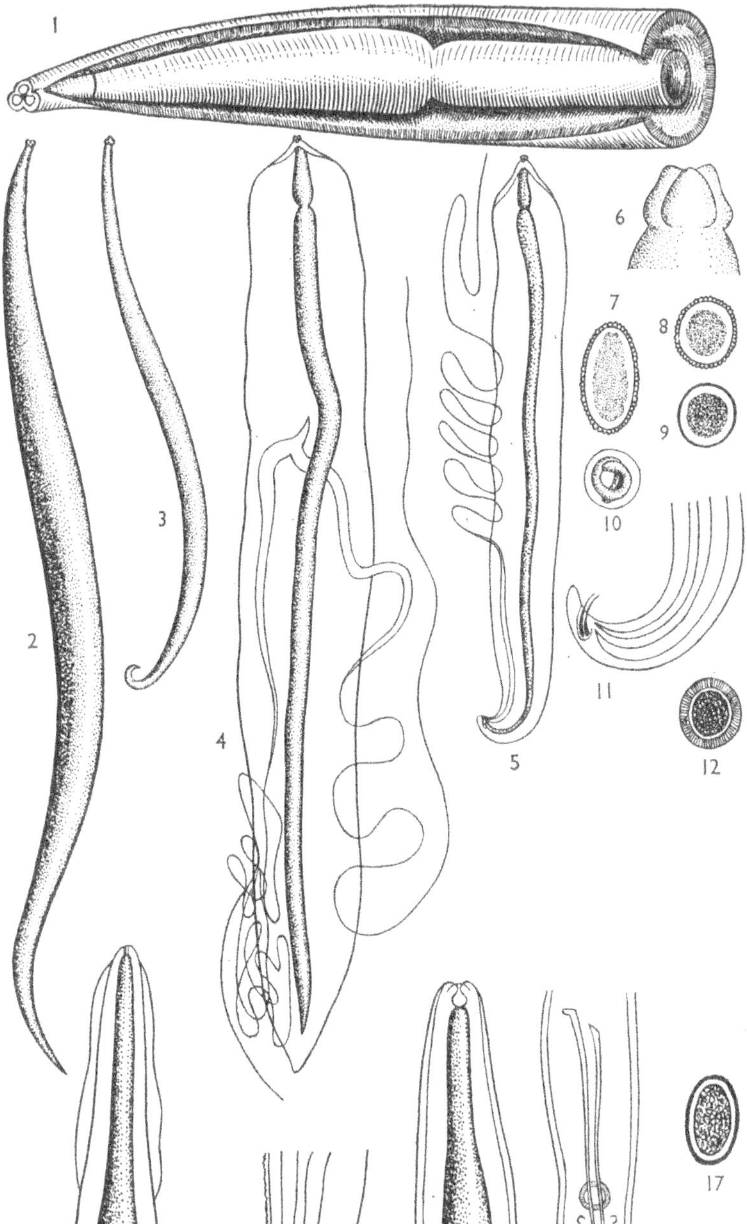
1
2
3
4
5
6
7
8
9
10
11
12
13
14
15
16
17

before they reach the infective stage. If they are then swallowed they hatch in the duodenum, liberating second-stage juveniles which penetrate the intestinal mucosa and are carried through the venous or lymphatic circulation to the heart and lungs. Here they break out into the air-sacs; moult twice; and migrate up the respiratory tree and down through the oesophagus and stomach to reach the intestine again, where the final moult is undergone and maturity achieved. There are no known reservoir hosts, although a physiological race of the parasite (not transmissible to man) occurs in the pig. Man acquires the infection by the ingestion of infective eggs in food or drink or on contaminated hands. In heavy infections the larval migration phase is associated with lobular pneumonitis, pulmonary consolidation and bronchial irritation, with resulting cough, haemoptysis and dyspnoea. The adults, if numerous, produce such toxaemic effects as fever, sweating, urticaria, asthma, insomnia and irritability. Traumatic damage with associated symptoms may result from intestinal obstruction by masses of adult worms; or from obstruction of the appendiceal lumen, the bile duct or the pancreatic duct, or from perforation of the intestinal wall by single individuals. Dramatic symptoms are sometimes produced when either adults or migrating juveniles reach unusual situations in the body.

Related species normally parasitic in dogs (*Toxocara canis*) and cats (*Toxocara cati*) occasionally infect man as adults. More frequently their juveniles, in attempting to establish themselves in the human body, produce a syndrome known as **visceral larva migrans,**

FIG. 15. Ascaroid Parasites

1 *Ascaris lumbricoides*—anterior end of adult worm, opened laterally to show nerve-ring, pharynx and intestine.
2 —adult female.
3 —adult male.
4 —adult female, opened mid-dorsally to show alimentary canal and partially unravelled paired ovaries and female ducts.
5 —adult male, opened mid-dorsally, to show alimentary canal and unravelled single testis and male ducts.
6 —dorsal view of anterior extremity, showing lips.
7 —unfertilised egg.
8 —normal fertilised egg.
9 —decorticated egg.
10 —embryonated egg.
11 —posterior extremity of adult male, showing spicules (side view).
12 *Toxocara canis*—egg.
13 —anterior extremity of adult worm, showing cervical alae.
14 —posterior extremity of male worm, showing spicules (side view).
15 *Ascaridia galli*—anterior end of adult worm.
16 —posterior end of male worm, showing caudal alae, papillae and spicules.
17 —egg.

the most conspicuous symptom of which is respiratory distress due to pulmonary infiltration, but which may manifest itself in a variety of other ways according to the location reached by the worms, including blindness if they penetrate the eye.

A number of ascarid species infect domestic animals, some of which may be of considerable veterinary importance. These include:

Neoascaris vitulorum in cattle,
Parascaris equorum in equines,
Ascaris columnaris in fur-bearers,
Toxascaris leonina in dogs, cats and foxes,
Toxocara canis in dogs and foxes,
Toxocara cati in cats,
Ascaridia galli in fowls, guinea-fowls, turkeys and geese,
Ascaridia columbae in pigeons,
Porrocaecum crassum in ducks; it requires an intermediate host, the juveniles encysting in the intermuscular connective tissue of fish.

Intra-uterine infection of offspring can occur prenatally from a mother animal infected with *Neoascaris vitulorum* or *Toxocara canis*. Diarrhoea, colic, anaemia, emaciation, a staring coat and restlessness are usual symptoms. In poultry egg-production is decreased. In canines pot-belly may be conspicuous. Heavy infections in any host may be serious.

In the treatment of human ascarid infection, dithiazanine and bephenium hydroxynaphthoate are the drugs of choice; but piperazine salts, diethylcarbamazine and hexylresorcinol can also be effectively employed. In animal infections all these drugs are used, and in addition sodium fluoride, phenothiazine, hygromycin B, cadmium oxide, carbon tetrachloride, carbon disulphide, toluene, oil of chenopodium (and the extract known as ascaridol). In poultry piperazine, dibutyl tin dilaurate with phenothiazine and nicotine, and penicillin and other antibiotics have been employed with success.

Prevention of human ascarid infection is primarily a matter of sanitary disposal of faeces and personal cleanliness and hygiene. No unwashed salads or raw vegetables should be consumed, especially if unsterilized night soil has been used in their cultivation. Prevention of animal infection is difficult and the most that can be done is to ensure the most meticulous cleanliness of pig styes, poultry pens and houses, stables and byres.

Strongyloidea

Two species of this order, *Ancylostoma duodenale* and *Necator americanus*, the notorious **hookworms** or **assassin worms,** are human parasites of major importance. Since they have similar life-cycles and produce identical syndromes, it will be convenient to consider them together:

Ancylostoma duodenale; Necator americanus. The present-day distribution of these two species involves much overlapping, having been complicated by population movements from infected areas. *A. duodenale* was probably originally endemic north of the Tropic of Cancer, around the Mediterranean Sea, and in India, China and Japan. *N. americanus*, on the other hand, was probably originally confined to areas south of the Tropic of Cancer in Africa, and to Southern Asia, the East Indies and the Pacific Islands. Each species remains dominant in the original area of its endemicity, while *N. americanus* is dominant in the western hemisphere, where it was carried by infected African slaves. Both species are small (5–13 by 0·3–0·6 mm), fusiform worms, the female being somewhat larger than the male. The cervical region is flexed, smoothly in *A. duodenale* and sharply in *N. americanus*—hence the name 'Hookworm'. The buccal capsule of *A. duodenale* is provided with teeth, while that of *N. americanus* is furnished with cutting plates. The males possess a copulatory bursa posteriorly, in which the arrangement of the supporting rays differs in the two species.

The adult worms occur in the small intestine, attached to the mucosa by the buccal capsule. They feed by sucking blood from lacerated capillary vessels. The eggs pass out in the faeces and hatch in the soil, giving rise to free-living, rhabditiform juveniles which feed on bacteria and, after moulting twice, change into non-feeding, infective, filariform juveniles. These latter await an opportunity to penetrate the human skin, reach a capillary vessel and be carried by the blood through the heart to the lungs. Here they break out into the air-sacs and migrate up the respiratory tree and down through the oesophagus and stomach, moulting *en route*, to reach maturity following a final moult in the intestine. Man acquires the infection by walking barefoot on infected soil. Except for limited foci in mines in Europe and elsewhere, these worms are confined to the warmer regions of the world (30° S latitude to 30° N latitude) by the fact that the free-living juveniles require a warm soil temperature in order to complete their development to the infective stage. There are no known reservoir hosts. The pathogenic effects are threefold:

(*a*) The invading filariform juveniles may produce a parasitic dermatitis, more severe in sensitised persons.

(*b*) The migration of juveniles through the lungs may be symptomless, but is often marked by cough, sore throat, hoarseness and haemoptysis. In heavy infections lobular consolidation and pneumonitis occur.

(*c*) The adults provoke intestinal haemorrhage and chronic enteritis, in addition to the heavy blood losses which they cause in feeding. Secondary, microcytic, hypochromic anaemia of haemorrhagic origin is usually present and may be very severe in heavy infections, with haemoglobin levels as low as 15 per cent and erythrocyte counts below 1,000,000 per cubic millimetre. Secondary changes in the vasoformative tissues, myocarditis, and degenerative hepatic changes may occur in severe cases. The picture is often complicated by chronic malnutrition.

Related species normally parasitic in cats and dogs (*Ancylostoma braziliense*, *A. caninum* and *Uncinaria stenocephala*) and cattle (*Bunostomum phlebotomum*) sometimes produce a pruritic skin lesion due to the abortive efforts of the infective juveniles tunnelling in the stratum germinativum to penetrate deeper. This infection, which is widespread in the warmer parts of the world, is contracted by man by contact with soil or pastures where the infected definitive hosts have defaecated. Children are the most frequent sufferers.

A large number of members of this order are of veterinary importance, the following among them:

Strongylus equinus, *S. edentatus* and *S. vulgaris* in the caecum and colon of equines which are commonly known as the 'large strongyles'.

Triodontophorus spp. and *Craterostomum* spp. in the caecum and colon of equines which are commonly known as the 'small strongyles'.

Cyathostomum spp. and *Cylicostomum* spp. (*Trichonema* spp.) and *Poteriostomum* spp. in the large intestine of equines.

In some of these species (e.g. trichonemids and *S. equinus*) the larvae develop in nodules in the intestinal wall. Mixed infections are the rule and it is therefore difficult to attribute specific pathogenic effects to any one species. All the horse strongyles attach themselves to the mucosa like hookworms and many suck blood. Young animals suffer most from infection. Diarrhoea, anaemia, emaciation and rough coat are the usual symptoms in severe cases.

Codiostomum struthionis is a dangerously pathogenic parasite which occurs in the large intestine of the ostrich.

Bourgelatia diducta occurs in the caecum and colon of the pig in India and South-East Asia. Little is known of its pathogenicity.

Oesophagostomum columbianum, *Oe. venulosum* and *Oe. asperum* occur in the colon of sheep, goats and camels, producing inflammatory nodules in the intestinal wall with resulting diarrhoea, exhaustion and death.

Oe. radiatum occurs similarly in cattle and *Oe. dentatum* in pigs.

Chabertia ovina occurs in the colon of sheep, goats and cattle, attaching itself to the mucosa, sucking blood and causing colitis, anaemia and even death.

Stephanurus dentatus occurs in the kidney, ureters and peri-renal region of pigs causing local and hepatic lesions.

Syngamus trachea (the **Gapeworm**) occurs in the trachea of turkeys, fowls, geese and various other birds, domestic and wild, sucking blood and causing tracheitis, cough and dyspnoea.

S. laryngeus occurs in the larynx of cattle in South America and Southern Asia, and *S. nasicola* in the nasal cavities of sheep, cattle and goats in various parts of the world.

Cyathostoma bronchialis infects the trachea and bronchi of ducks, geese and swans, producing dyspnoea and asphyxiation, especially in young birds.

Ancylostoma caninum and *A. braziliense*, already referred to above, occur as adults in the small intestine of dogs, cats and some furbearers.

Agriostomum vryburgi occurs in the small intestine of cattle in India and South-East Asia.

Necator suillus occurs in the small intestine of pigs in Trinidad.

Bunostomum trigonocephalum occurs in the small intestine of sheep and goats.

B. phlebotomum is found similarly in cattle.

Gaigeria pachyscelis occurs in the small intestine of sheep and goats in India and Africa.

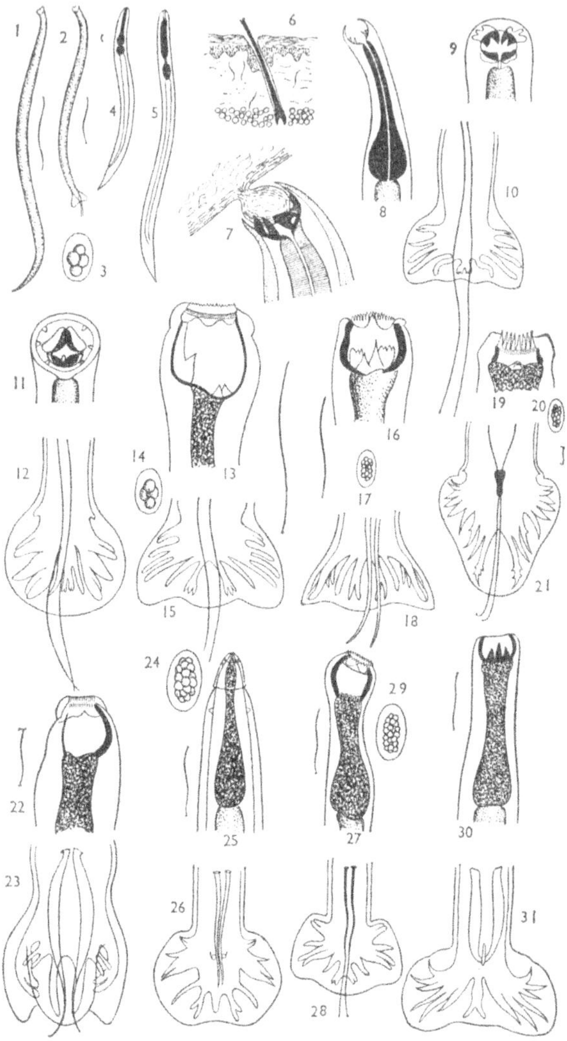

FIG. 16. Hookworms

1 Human Hookworm—adult female.
2 —adult male.
3 —egg.
4 —rhabditiform (first-stage) juvenile.
5 —filariform (second-stage or infective) juvenile.
6 —filariform larva penetrating skin.
7 —section of anterior end of adult worm attached to intestinal wall and grasping a plug of mucosa in its buccal capsule.
8 —anterior end of adult worm to show shape of oesophagus.
9 *Ancylostoma duodenale*—head and buccal capsule in ventral view, showing teeth.
10 —posterior end of male, showing copulatory bursa and spicules.
11, 12 *Necator americanus*—head and buccal capsule in ventral view, showing cutting plates.

Globocephalus spp. occurs in the small intestine of the pig, especially in eastern countries.

Uncinaria stenocephala in the small intestine of dogs, cats and fur-bearers, has been referred to above.

Amidostomum anseris (*A. nodulosum*) occurs in the gizzard, proventriculus and oesophagus of geese and ducks, burrowing in the mucosa and submucosa.

Since the majority of strongyloid worms enter the host through the skin, migrate through the lungs as juveniles and suck blood from the vessels in the wall of the alimentary tract as adults, causing some degree of irritation, inflammation and haemorrhage in each location, they normally cause a sequence of cutaneous, pulmonary and systemic symptoms, which vary in severity according to the number of worms present. Anaemia, weakness and loss of condition, diarrhoea, and emaciation are commonly observed in all these infections.

Dithiazanine and bephenium hydroxynaphthoate have been found to be highly effective in the treatment of human hookworm infection, and are now the drugs of choice. Tetrachlorethylene, hexylresorcinol and carbon tetrachloride, which were formerly used, are now falling into disrepute on account of their lesser efficacy and greater side-effects. In animal infections piperazine and phenothiazine have largely replaced carbon tetrachloride and oil of chenopodium; but there are signs that phenothiazine-resistant

---

13 *Strongylus equinus*—anterior end of adult worm, showing buccal capsule in side view.
14 —egg.
15 —posterior end of male, showing copulatory bursa and spicules.
16 *Triodontophorus serratus*—anterior end of adult worm, showing buccal capsule in side view.
17 —egg.
18 —posterior end of male, showing copulatory bursa and spicules.
19 *Trichonema aegyptiacum*—anterior end of adult-worm, showing buccal capsule in side view.
20 —egg.
21 —posterior end of male, showing copulatory bursa and spicules.
22 *Codiostomum struthionis*—anterior end of adult worm, showing buccal capsule in side view.
23 —posterior end of male, showing copulatory bursa and spicules.
24 *Oesophagostomum columbianum*—anterior end of adult worm.
25 —egg.
26 —posterior end of male worm, showing copulatory bursa and spicules.
27 *Chabertia ovina*—anterior end of adult worm, showing buccal capsule in side view.
28 —posterior end of male, showing copulatory bursa and spicules.
29 —egg.
30 *Amidostomum anseris*—anterior end of adult worm, showing buccal capsule.
31 —posterior end of male, showing copulatory bursa and spicules.

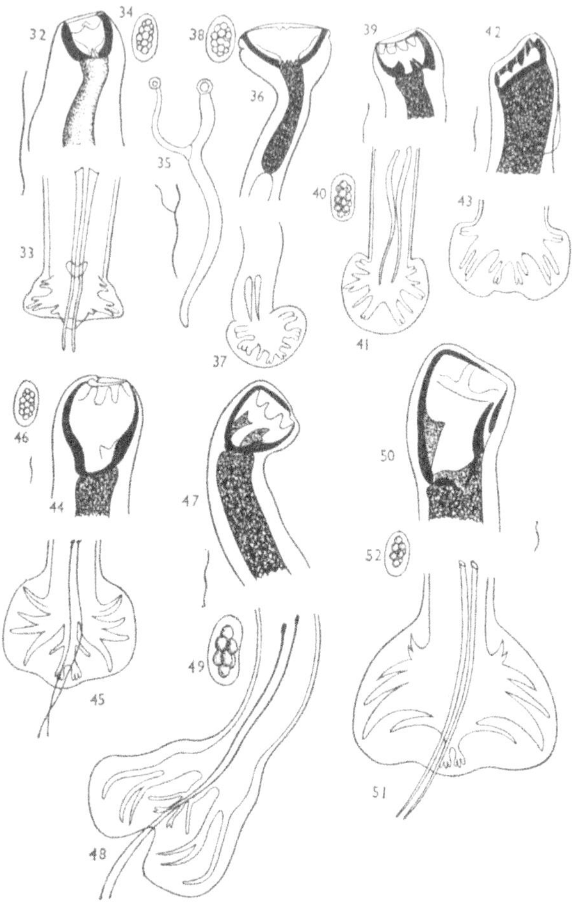

FIG. 16. Hookworms (*continued*)

32 *Stephanurus dentatus*—anterior end of adult worm, showing buccal capsule in side view.
33 —posterior end of male, showing copulatory bursa and spicules.
34 —egg.
35 *Syngamus trachea*—male and female worms *in copulo*.
36 —anterior end of adult worm, showing buccal capsule.
37 —posterior end of male worm, showing copulatory bursa and spicules.
38 —egg.
39 *Gaigeria pachyscelis*—anterior end of adult worm, showing buccal capsule in side view.
40 —egg.
41 —posterior end of male, showing copulatory bursa and spicules.
42 *Agriostomum vryburgi*—anterior end of adult worm, showing buccal capsule in side view.
43 —posterior end of male, showing copulatory bursa.
44 *Globocephalus urosubulatus*—anterior end of adult worm, showing buccal capsule in side view.
45 —posterior end of male, showing copulatory bursa and spicules.
46 —egg.

races of strongyloid parasites are developing. Hygromycin B has also been found to be effective, and has been used with success prophylactically by adding small doses to the food. *Syngamus* spp. are effectively treated with barium antimony tartrate. Against infection with *Stephanurus dentatus* there is, as yet, no satisfactory treatment. An iron tonic is beneficial in the treatment of all forms of infection with strongyloid worms in order to counteract the anaemia resulting from their blood-sucking activities.

Prevention of human hookworm infection involves sanitary disposal of faeces, prevention of promiscuous defaecation, avoidance of the use of night-soil as a fertiliser or its sterilisation before application, and mass treatment of all human cases. The wearing of foot-gear, sometimes advocated, while admittedly effective as a prophylactic measure, is not practicable under the circumstances existing in most endemic areas; it does not, in any case, prevent infection in mines, where the infective juveniles are transferred on the boots of the miners to the rungs of ladders which they will subsequently grasp with their bare hands. Frequent spraying with lysol is a useful measure in mines. Ploughing-in of lethal dusts, such as lime, ammonium sulphate or sodium nitrate not only kills the juveniles in the soil but also improves fertility. Against animal infection pasture rotation is the most important measure.

Trichostrongyloidea

At least seven species of the genus *Trichostrongylus*, normally parasitic in herbivorous animals (sheep, goats, camels, equines, rabbits, deer and antelopes) are not uncommon as human parasites. The adults are small (5–9 mm), slender, reddish worms which inhabit the stomach and anterior part of the small intestine. Human infection is most frequent in the Far East (Japan, Korea and Indonesia), but is also relatively common in parts of the U.S.S.R., South and South-East Asia, Australia, Africa, the Middle East and Chile. The life-cycle of these worms is similar to that of the human hookworms, the eggs being voided in the faeces and passing

47 *Bunostomum phlebotomum*—anterior end of adult worm, showing buccal capsule in side view.
48 —posterior end of male, showing copulatory bursa and spicules.
49 —egg.
50 *Uncinaria stenocephala*—anterior end of adult worm, showing buccal capsule in side view.
51 —posterior end of male, showing copulatory bursa and spicules.
52 —egg.

through a free-living juvenile phase in the soil. The infective juvenile, although capable of entering the body through the skin, normally climbs onto a grass blade and is ingested by the definitive host with its food. In man infection is invariably acquired by the oral route as, for example, by sucking contaminated grass stalks, ingesting contaminated green-stuff, or via oral contact with contaminated hands. Human infection is generally light and symptomless; but heavy infections with mucosal desquamation, mild secondary anaemia, dry skin and emaciation, sometimes occur.

Trichostrongylosis is much more important as a veterinary problem. The following species infect domestic animals:

Trichostrongylus spp. in sheep, goats, camels, equines, rabbits and cattle—mainly in the small intestine.

Graphidium strigosum in the stomach and small intestine of rabbits in Europe.

Ostertagia spp. and *Marshallagia* spp. in the abomasum of sheep, goats and cattle.

Cooperia spp. in the small intestine of cattle, sheep and goats.

Nematodirus spp. in the small intestine of cattle, sheep and goats.

Haemonchus spp. in the stomach and intestine of cattle, sheep and goats and other ruminants, generally inhabit the abomasum and are known as wireworms or stomach worms. They are seriously pathogenic.

Mecistocirrus digitatus occurs in the abomasum of sheep and cattle and in the stomach of pigs in eastern countries and Central America.

Ollulanus tricuspis occurs in the stomach of cats, fur-bearers and occasionally pigs and is transmitted by the ingestion of vomit. It is viviparous.

Hyostrongylus rubidus in the stomach of pigs.

Ornithostrongylus quadriradiatus in the crop, proventriculus and small intestine of pigeons in North America, South Africa and Australia.

Libyostrongylus douglassii in the proventriculus of ostriches in South Africa.

Anaemia, weakness, emaciation and stunting are common effects of heavy infection with any of these worms. Diarrhoea or constipation, often with dark faeces, and a dry, harsh coat are also frequently observed. Some species are more pathogenic than others

Trichostrongylosis is much more of a veterinary than a medical problem, since human infections rarely show serious symptoms. The worms are refractory to most forms of treatment, but piperazine salts are said to have some effect and bephenium hydroxynaphthoate is now being used. Formerly hexylresorcinol and tetrachlorethylene were the drugs of choice. In animal infections toluene, tetrachlorethylene, various organophosphorus compounds and a number of bephenium salts (hydroxynaphthoate, naphthoate, bromide, chloride and iodide) are used; but two new drugs recently introduced show remarkable promise, namely, methydrine (2-(β-methoxyethyl)-pyridine) and thiabendazole (2-(4′-thiazolyl-benzimidadzole), the former being administered by subcutaneous injection and the latter orally. These two drugs are also said to be effective against ascarids, trichurids, and *Strongyloides* spp. in domestic animals.

Prevention of trichostrongylosis in man is a simple matter of avoiding oral contact with anything which may carry or may have been in contact with anything carrying the infective juveniles. This means principally avoiding chewing or sucking pieces of grass, but should also mean a ban on oral contact with dirty hands. The prevention of infection in domestic animals is more difficult. Resistance to infection should be kept high by good feeding and the provision of mineral licks to correct deficiencies. Infected beasts should be treated. Overstocking should be avoided. Young animals should be separated from their mothers as soon as weaned, since they are more susceptible. Wet pastures should not be used; and stabled animals should be fed from raised troughs.

Metastrongyloidea

Members of this order rarely infect man, but the cosmopolitan species *Metastrongylus apri* is an important parasite of pigs and less frequently occurs in cattle and sheep. The adult worm inhabits the bronchi and bronchioles, often causing severe bronchitis, which may be fatal. The eggs are coughed up and pass out of the definitive host in the sputum or faeces. They hatch in the soil. The juveniles must, however, be ingested by a suitable species of earthworm, in which development to the infective stage takes place. The definitive host becomes infected by eating the infected earthworm. A few cases of human infection have been reported.

A number of species belonging to this order are of veterinary importance, among them:

Dictyocaulus filaria, which occurs in the bronchi of sheep and goats and has no intermediate host, the infective juveniles being ingested by the definitive host.

D. viviparus, which occurs in the bronchi of cattle, causing the syndrome known as 'husk' or 'hoose' characterised by catarrhal bronchitis, dyspnoea, cough, diarrhoea, anaemia and emaciation and often terminating in secondary pneumonia.

Protostrongylus spp., which occur in the small bronchioles of sheep and goats and cause lobar pneumonia. An intermediate host is required—the land snail *Helicella*.

Cystocaulus ocreatus also occurs in the small bronchioles of sheep and requires an intermediate host—in this case the field slug *Agriolimax* or the land snail *Monacha*.

Metastrongylus spp. Several other species of this genus, in addition to *M. apri* (see above) occur in pigs. In addition to causing bronchitis and pneumonia, they transmit the virus of swine influenza.

Muellerius capillaris occurs in the lungs of sheep and goats, causing nodular pulmonary inflammation but not usually giving rise to symptoms. Slugs and land snails serve as intermediate hosts.

Aelurostrongylus abstrusus occurs in the lungs of cats, giving rise to pneumonitis with cough, diarrhoea and emaciation. Slugs and snails serve as intermediate hosts.

Angiostrongylus vasorum occurs in the pulmonary artery and right ventricle of dogs and fur-bearers. The intermediate hosts are unknown. This is a highly pathogenic parasite, since it blocks the branches of the pulmonary artery and so leads to perivascular sclerosis and pulmonary emphysema which, in turn, lead to cardiac hypertrophy and insufficiency. Liver changes with resulting ascites, and dyspnoea, also supervene.

Filarioides osleri occurs in the trachea and bronchi of dogs, causing cough, bronchitis and emaciation. The intermediate hosts are unknown.

Crenosoma vulpis occurs in the bronchi of foxes and other fur-bearers, causing bronchitis and pneumonia. Land snails and slugs serve as intermediate hosts.

None of the many methods of treatment advocated in the past has been really effective, and much remains to be learned in this

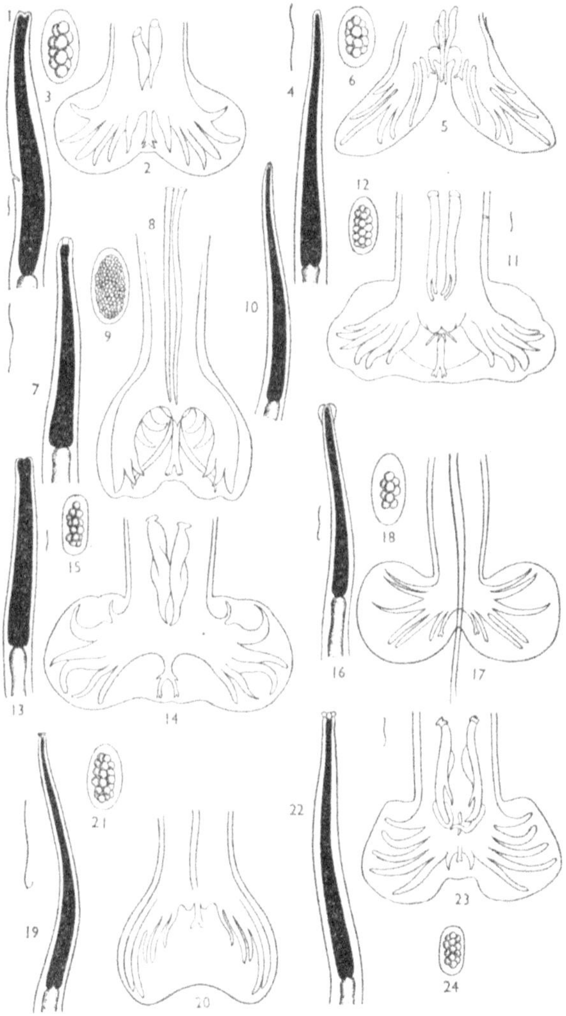

FIG. 17. Trichostrongyloid Worms

1 *Trichostrongylus colubriformis*—anterior end of adult worm.
2 —copulatory bursa and spicules of male.
3 —egg.
4 *Haemonchus contortus*—anterior end of adult worm.
5 —copulatory bursa and spicules of male.
6 —egg.
7 *Graphidium strigosum*—anterior end of adult worm.
8 —copulatory bursa and spicules of male.
9 —egg.
10 *Ostertagia ostertagi*—anterior end of adult worm.
11 —copulatory bursa and spicules of male.
12 —egg.
13 *Cooperia curticei*—anterior end of adult worm.
14 —copulatory bursa and spicules of male.
15 —egg.

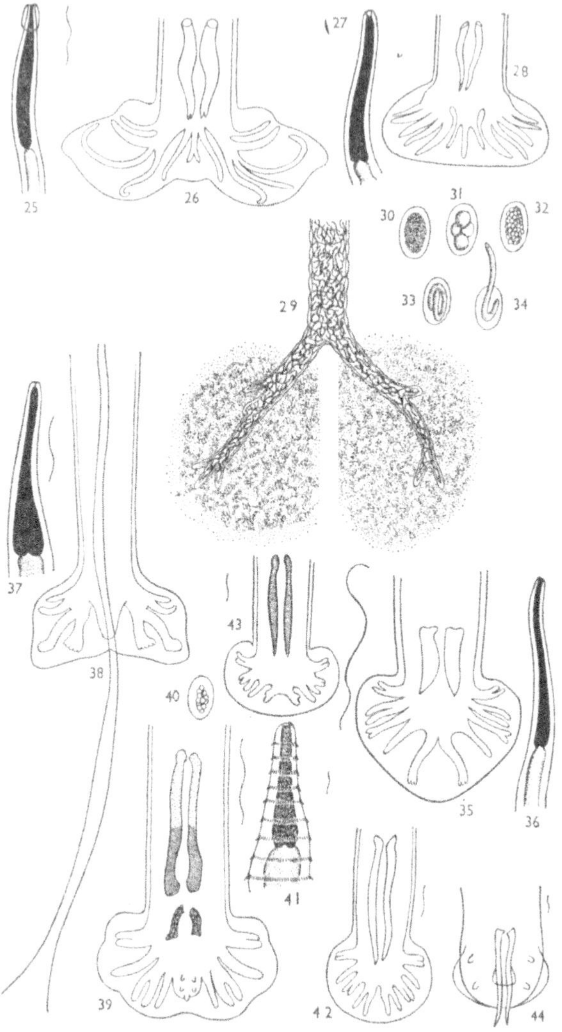

FIG. 17 (continued)

16 *Nematodirus filicollis*—anterior end of adult worm.
17 —copulatory bursa and spicules of male.
18 —egg.
19 *Mecistocirrus digitatus*—anterior end of adult worm.
20 —copulatory bursa and spicules of male.
21 —egg.
22 *Hyostrongylus rubidus*—anterior end of adult worm.
23 —copulatory bursa and spicules of male.
24 —egg.
25 *Ornithostrongylus quadriradiatus*—anterior end of adult worm.
26 —copulatory bursa and spicules of male.
27 *Ollulanus tricuspis*—anterior end of adult worm.
28 —copulatory bursa and spicules of male.

field. The relatively new drug cyanacethydrazide (Dictycide, Helmox) has, however, shown great promise in the treatment of ungulates, and trivalent antimonials have been beneficial in the treatment of cats, dogs and fur-bearers.

Dry pastures are, perhaps, the most important single measure in the avoidance of metastrongyloid infections in grazing animals. Vaccination with irradiated juveniles was introduced a few years ago as a preventive measure against *Dictyocaulus* infection in cattle and was at first hailed as a success. Further experience with the method, however, has raised doubts, in particular as to the duration of the immunity, especially in the absence of exposure to re-infection; and vaccinated animals have been claimed to act as carriers and therefore to be a danger to other stock.

Spiruroidea

Members of this order occur in man only occasionally as accidental parasites. The species most frequently found is *Gongylonema pulchrum.*

Gongylonema pulchrum. This is a cosmopolitan form, normally parasitic in pigs, wild and domestic ungulates, and monkeys. The adults, which may reach 15 by 0·5 cm, burrow in the mucosa and submucosa of the buccal cavity, tongue and pharynx, causing local irritation. The eggs pass out in the faeces and hatch if ingested by dung-beetles or cockroaches. Man acquires the infection by accidental ingestion of insects containing the infective stage.

A number of spiruroids are of importance in veterinary medicine. All of them are partially or entirely tissue-parasites, burrowing in the walls of the organs they inhabit. Table 9 indicates the principal ones.

Spiruroid infections are notoriously difficult to treat, owing to the habit of the worms of burrowing in the mucosa or of forming nodules. However, both carbon disulphide and diethylcarbamazine

---

29 *Dictyocaulus filaria*—trachea, bronchi and lungs of infected sheep, showing adult worms in air-passages.
30/34 —eggs, showing stages in development and hatching of larva.
35 —copulatoty bursa and spicules of male.
36 —anterior end of adult worm.
37 *Metastrongylus apri*—anterior end of adult worm.
38 —copulatory bursa and spicules of male worm.
39 *Protostrongylus rufescens*—copulatory bursa and spicules of male worm.
40 —egg.
41 *Crenosoma vulpis*—anterior end of adult worm.
42 —copulatory bursa and spicules of male worm.
43 *Aelurostrongylus abstrusus*—copulatory bursa and spicules of male worm.
44 *Filarioides osleri*—copulatory bursa and spicules of male worm.

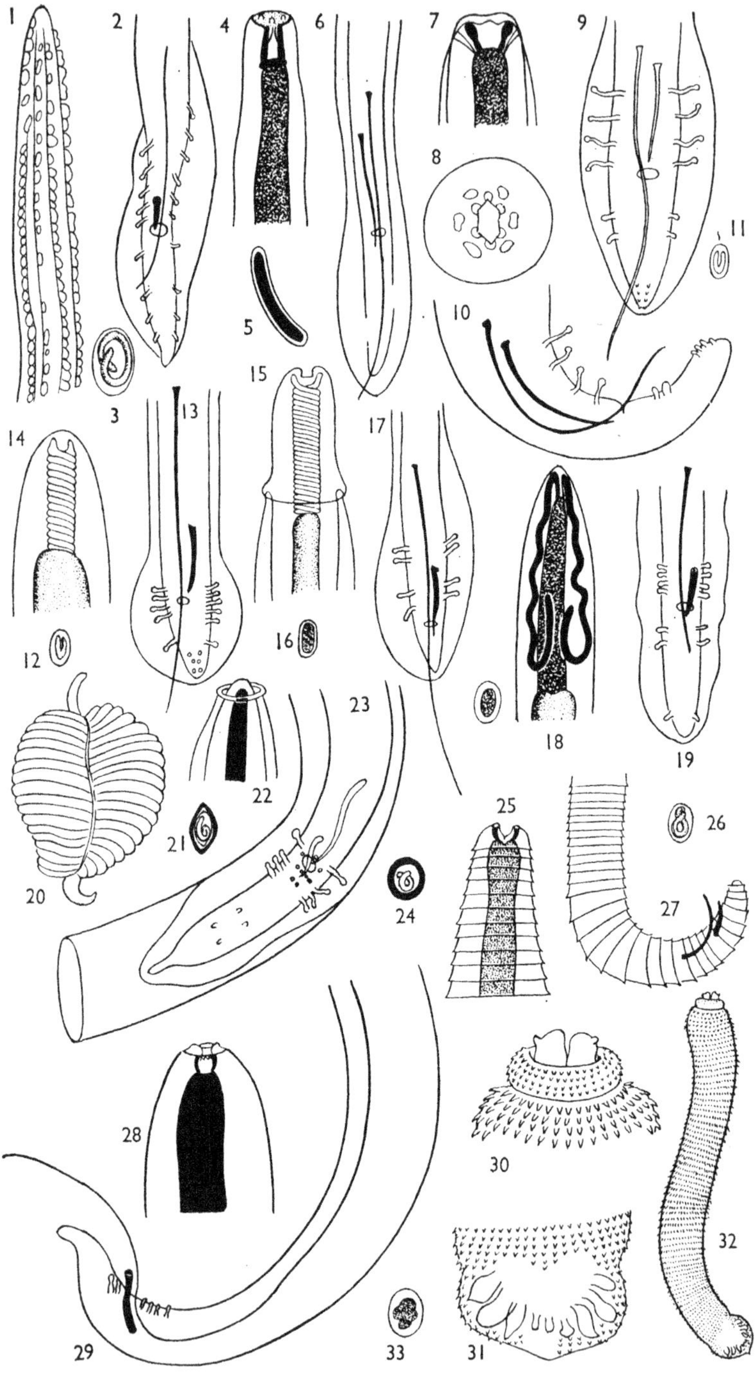
1
2
3
4
5
6
7
8
9
10
11
12
13
14
15
16
17
18
19
20
21
22
23
24
25
26
27
28
29
30
31
32
33

are said to be effective provided that the gut is flushed with sodium bicarbonate solution before administration in order to loosen the mucus which surrounds the worms.

Prevention involves measures against the intermediate hosts and the hygienic disposal of manure.

Dracunculoidea

A single species of this order is parasitic in man.

Dracunculus medinensis **(the Guinea worm).** This species, which is believed to be the form referred to in the Pentateuch as the 'burning fiery serpent', is endemic in a wide belt stretching through North and Central Africa, Arabia and Southern Asia, and also in parts of Central and South America. The adult worms inhabit the deeper

---

FIG. 18. Spiruroidea Worms

1 *Gongylonema pulchrum*—anterior end of adult worm showing bosses.
2 —posterior end of male, showing caudal papillae, spicules and alae.
3 —egg.
4 *Habronema microstoma*—anterior end of adult worm, showing vestibule.
5 —egg.
6 —posterior end of male, showing caudal papillae, alae and spicules.
7 *Spirocerca lupi*—anterior end of adult worm, showing vestibule.
8 —front view of head, showing trilobed lips.
9 —posterior end of male, showing caudal papillae, alae and spicules.
10 —posterior end of male in side view.
11 —egg.
12 *Ascarops strongulina*—egg.
13 —posterior end of male, showing caudal alae, papillae and spicules.
14 —anterior end of adult worm, showing characteristic pharynx.
15 *Physocephalus sexalatus*—anterior end of adult worm, showing characteristic pharynx.
16 —egg.
17 —posterior end of male, showing caudal alae, papillae and spicules.
18 *Acuaria spiralis*—anterior end of adult worm, showing cordons. Egg at side.
19 —posterior end of male worm, showing caudal alae, papillae and spicules.
20 *Tetrameres* sp.—subspherical female.
21 —egg.
22 *Physaloptera praeputialis*—anterior end of adult worm, showing collar.
23 —posterior end of male worm, showing caudal alae, papillae and spicules, and projecting cuticular sheath.
24 —egg.
25 *Thelazia rhodesii*—anterior end of adult worm showing vestibule and transverse cuticular striations.
26 —egg.
27 —posterior end of male, showing spicules and striations.
28 *Oxyspirura mansoni*—anterior end of adult worm, showing vestibule.
29 —posterior end of male, showing spicules and caudal papillae in side view.
30 *Gnathostoma spinigerum*—anterior end of adult worm, showing head-bulb armed with sharp spines and enclosing large fleshy lips, and flat body spines.
31 —posterior end of male, showing caudal papillae and spines.
32 —entire adult male.
33 —egg.

TABLE 9

Parasite	Definitive hosts	Location in hosts	Intermediate hosts	Pathogenic effects
Habronema spp.	Equines	Stomach	House-flies Stable-flies	Gastric tumours, summer sores (juveniles) catarrhal gastritis
Hartertia gallinarum	Fowls	Small intestine	Termites	Emaciation, weakness, diarrhoea (Africa)
Spirocerca spp.	Dogs, fur-bearers	Oesophagus, stomach, aorta	Dung-beetles	Interference with swallowing, breathing, circulation
Ascarops spp.	Pigs	Stomach	Dung-beetles	Gastritis, leading to loss of appetite, excessive thirst, retarded growth, emaciation
Physocephalus sexalatus	Pigs, rabbits	Stomach	Dung-beetles	
Simondsia paradoxa	Pigs	Stomach	Dung-beetles?	
Gongylonema spp.	Sheep, goats, cattle, pigs, equines, camels, fowls	Oesophagus, rumen, crop	Dung-beetles, cockroaches	Although some local irritation must be caused, these forms apparently produce no serious effects. although *G. neoplasticum* stimulates malignant growths in rats
Acuaria spp.	Fowls, turkeys, ducks, geese, swans, pigeons	Gizzard, oesophagus, proventriculus, small intestine	Arthropods: Grasshoppers, beetles, isopods, copepods	Weakened gizzard muscles due to nodules Toxic effects Emaciation, droopiness, weakness, anaemia
Tetrameres spp.	Fowls, turkeys, pigeons, ducks	Proventriculus	Orthoptera, e.g. cockroaches. Fresh-water crustacea, e.g. *Daphnia*, *Gammarus*	Local inflammation and irritation Toxic effects Fatal in chicks
Physaloptera spp.	Cats, dogs	Stomach	Beetles, cockroaches, crickets	Severe gastritis Loss of condition Heavy infections fatal
Thelazia spp.	Cattle, sheep, goats, equines	Eye, lacrimal ducts	House-flies (*Musca* spp.)	Conjunctivitis lacrimation, photophobia, ophthalmia, blindness
Oxyspirura spp.	Fowls, turkeys, peahens	Eye, lacrimal ducts	Cockroaches	
Gnathostoma spp.	Cats, dogs, fur-bearers pigs (man)	Stomach, liver (juveniles)	1. *Cyclops* 2. Fresh-water fish	Severe inflammation of affected organs Tumours filled with blood and pus Cachexia. Death (In man, juveniles occur under the skin, causing a form ofcreepingeruption)

subcutaneous tissues. The female is a long (50–100 cm), filiform worm, rarely exceeding one millimetre in thickness. The much smaller (2–4 cm) male is not often seen. After copulation the uterus of the viviparous female becomes filled with eggs, which hatch *in situ*. The female then migrates to the superficial subcutaneous tissues of the limbs, especially in the region of the legs and feet, and there gives rise, by means of a toxic exudate, to a small, shallow, perforate ulcer, through which she can protrude the anterior part of her body carrying the genital opening. When the ulcer comes into contact with water the female contracts convulsively, often rupturing the protruding portion of the body-wall and the uterus within it, and so discharging a cloud of juveniles into the water. The juveniles swim about until ingested by a suitable species of the small crustacean *Cyclops*, when they burrow through the intestinal wall into the body-cavity and there develop to the infective stage. If the *Cyclops* is then swallowed by a suitable definitive host the juvenile is liberated by digestion and migrates through the gut-wall and further tissues to reach the subcutaneous layers, where it develops to the adult stage. There are probably no natural reservoir hosts, but records of the occurrence of this species in domestic animals do exist. Man acquires the infection by accidental ingestion of ingested *Cyclops* while bathing, or through drinking unfiltered water. Multiple infection is common. Although the migration of the gravid female to skin level may produce generalised allergic and toxic symptoms in some cases, the principal effect of this parasite is in the production of the skin lesions, which first appear as itching, reddish papules, and then burst to form burning, painful ulcers.

A related species, *D. insignis*, occurs in dogs and fur-bearing mammals (foxes, skunks, weasels, raccoons and mink) in North America; but this species is apparently not transmissible to man.

Another related form, *Oshimaia taiwana*, occurs in ducks in Cochin China. Species of *Cyclops* again serve as intermediate hosts. The worms cause painful swelling under the mandible which interfere with swallowing and breathing and may even lead to death through asphyxia or inability to feed.

Removal of the female worms by traction or surgery is the only effective method of treatment in dracunculoid infections; but care must be taken not to break the parasite during the process as dangerous results may follow the release of its body-fluids into the system of sensitised animals or persons.

Prevention of human infection involves avoiding the drinking of unboiled or unfiltered water, and the treatment of infested water with lime, DDT or a mixture of copper sulphate and perchloron, to kill the intermediate hosts. The introduction of *Cyclops*-eating fish, such as *Barbus puckelli*, has also been advocated.

Filarioidea

Six species of this order are regularly parasitic in man.

Wuchereria bancrofti (**Bancroft's filaria).** This species is indigenous throughout the warmer regions of the globe in a broad belt extending from 30° N to 30° S in the western hemisphere and from 41° N to 28° S in the eastern hemisphere. It is hyper-endemic in South-East Asia and the Polynesian Islands. The adults are long, filiform worms, the female (8–10 cm by 0·25 mm) being larger than the male (4 cm by 0·1 mm). They inhabit the lymph-glands and lymphatic vessels. After copulation the viviparous female sheds active first-stage juveniles (microfilariae) which are enclosed by a flexible sheath representing the egg-membranes. The microfilariae find themselves in the circulation and usually show nocturnal periodicity, appearing in the peripheral blood at night but returning during the day to the capillaries of the lungs and other viscera. The intermediate host is a blood-sucking female mosquito, usually a night-biting form, within which the microfilariae imbibed with the blood-meal shed their sheath, penetrate the gut-wall and migrate to the thoracic musculature. Here they develop into infective third-stage juveniles which make their way forwards to the salivary glands and there await the opportunity of injection into a new definitive host individual. Man acquires the infection through the bites of infected mosquitoes. There are no known reservoir hosts. The microfilariae are non-pathogenic, but the adult worms provoke inflammatory and obstructive changes, particularly in the lymph glands. The inflammation results in toxaemia, fever and local pain. Obstruction of the lymph channels results in stagnation of the lymph and dilatation of the vessels with following hypertrophy and fibrosis of the affected tissues, leading eventually to elephantiasis, especially of the limbs, scrotum and mammae.

Brugia malayi. This species is closely related to *W. bancrofti*, which it resembles in most respects. However, the adult worms are somewhat smaller (2–5·5 cm by 0·1–0·2 mm); the parasite is found only in South-East Asia; the microfilariae differ slightly in appearance, being less smoothly curved in outline; and the elephantic lesions are more frequent in the upper limbs and are rarely observed in the lower limbs or scrotum. Both adults and microfilariae show anatomical differences in the two forms. Related species of the genus *Brugia* occur in dogs and cats. The intermediate hosts of *Brugia* are also mosquitoes.

Onchocerca volvulus (**the blinding filaria**). This species occurs in equatorial Africa, with the exception of the east coast; and in Guatemala and Southern Mexico. The adults are long filiform worms, the female being markedly larger (30–50 cm by 0·3–0·4 mm) than the male (2–4 cm by 0·1–0·2 mm). They inhabit the subcutaneous tissues, their presence giving rise to local inflammatory reaction and fibrotic nodules, each of which generally contains a male and a female worm. The viviparous female gives birth to unsheathed microfilariae which remain in the vicinity of the parent nodule, occupying the tissue- and lymph-spaces of the skin and peripheral connective tissue. The intermediate host is a species of black-fly belonging to the genus *Simulium*, within which the juvenile undergoes a similar sequence of development to that of *W. bancrofti* in the mosquito. Man acquires the infection through the bites of infected black-flies. The characteristic nodules, which may be numerous, are not usually painful unless situated over a joint; but they may be intensely pruritic. Much more serious are the ocular lesions which result from invasion of the eye by microfilariae and their death therein, giving rise to inflammatory reaction. Blindness not infrequently follows. Several related species occur in domestic animals (see Table 10 below).

Loa loa (**the eye worm**). This species is indigenous in Central and West Africa. The filariform adults range in size from 3 to 7 cm by 0·3 to 0·5 mm, the female being slightly larger than the male. They lead a migratory existence in the subcutaneous tissue, the viviparous female giving rise to sheathed microfilariae which circulate in the peripheral blood with a diurnal periodicity. *L. loa* is transmitted by the blood-sucking deer-flies of the genus *Chrysops*, within which the microfilariae undergo development to the infective stage. Certain species of monkeys act as reservoir hosts. Man acquires the infection through the bites of infected deer-flies. Temporary inflammatory swellings (**Calabar** or **fugitive swellings**) are provoked by the migratory adults. They cause pain and inconvenience, especially when in the neighbourhood of the eyes or the bridge of the nose.

Acanthocheilonema perstans. This species is widely distributed in

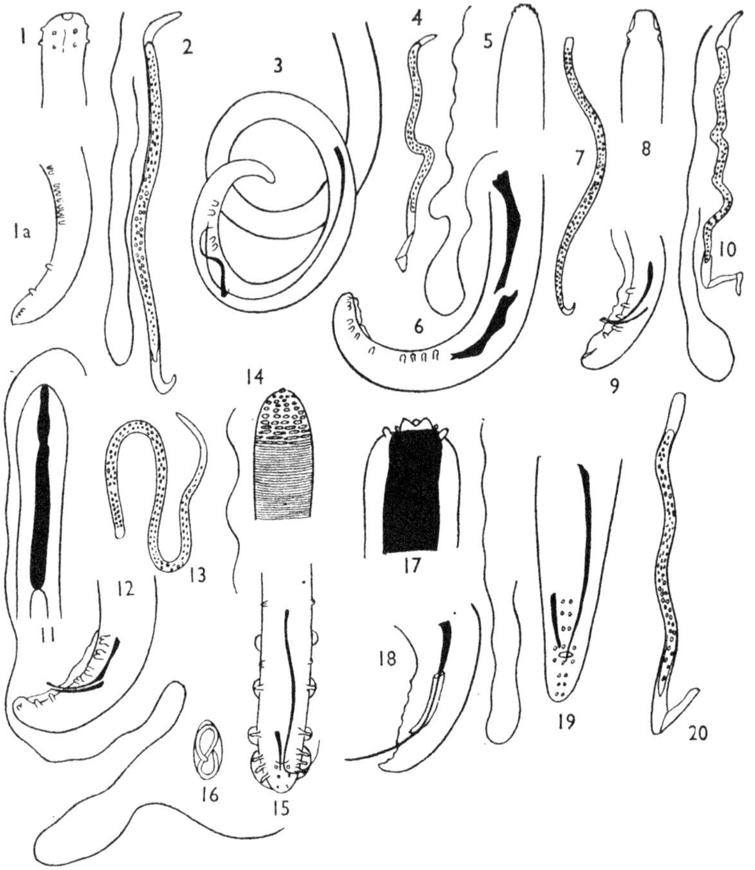

FIG. 19. Filarioid Worms

1 *Wuchereria bancrofti*—anterior end of adult worm.
1a —posterior end of male, showing caudal papillae (side view).
2 —microfilaria (sheathed).
3 *Brugia malayi*—posterior end of male, showing spiral coiling, caudal papillae and spicules (side view).
4 —microfilaria (sheathed).
5 *Onchocerca volvulus*—anterior end of adult worm.
6 —posterior end of male, showing caudal papillae and spicules (side view).
7 —microfilaria (unsheathed).
8 *Loa loa*—anterior end of adult worm.
9 —posterior end of male, showing caudal papillae and spicules (side view).
10 —microfilaria (sheathed).
11 *Dirofilaria immitis*—anterior end of adult worm.
12 —posterior end of male, showing caudal papillae and spicules (side view).
13 —microfilaria (unsheathed).
14 *Parafilaria multipapillosa*—anterior end of adult worm.
15 —posterior end of male, showing caudal papillae and spicules (ventral view).
16 —egg.
17 *Setaria equina*—anterior end of adult worm.
18 —posterior end of male, showing caudal papillae and spicules (side view).
19 —posterior end of male, showing caudal papillae and spicules (ventral view).
20 —microfilaria (sheathed).

the tropical areas of Africa and Central and South America. The adults, which are slightly larger than the adults of *L. loa*, inhabit the connective tissue of the mesenteries and the peritoneal cavity; more rarely they occur in the pericardial and pleural cavities. The viviparous female gives birth to unsheathed, aperiodic microfilariae, which circulate in the peripheral blood. The intermediate hosts are midges of the genus *Culicoides*. Certain other primates, including the chimpanzee and gorilla, act as reservoir hosts. Man acquires the infection through the bites of infected midges. The infection is essentially symptomless.

Mansonella ozzardi. This species occurs extensively in South America and the West Indian Islands. The adults, which are similar in size to those of *A. perstans*, occur free in the body cavity, threaded into the mesentery or embedded in the visceral adipose tissue. The viviparous female produces unsheathed aperiodic microfilariae, which circulate in the peripheral blood. Like *A. perstans*, the parasite is transmitted by midges of the genus *Culicoides*, through the bites of which man becomes infected. The infection is essentially symptomless.

A number of species of filariae infect domestic animals, as shown in Table 10.

The drugs which have been found to be most effective in the treatment of filarial infections in man are diethylcarbamazine, sodium thiacetarsamide and trivalent antimonials such as sodium antimony tartrate, and stibophen. These drugs are also used with effect in animal filariases, as is also dichlorophenarsine.

Prevention involves mass treatment of all infected persons or animals and strict measures against the intermediate hosts which transmit the infections.

Trichuroidea

Two very different parasites belonging to this order infect man.

Trichuris trichiura (**the whipworm**). This cosmopolitan species occurs most commonly in warm, moist climates. The adult worms are whip-shaped—narrow and thread-like anteriorly, broader and fusiform posteriorly—and range in length from 2 to 5 cm. They occur in the caecum and upper part of the colon, attached to the mucosa by their anterior ends. The eggs pass out in the faeces of the host and remain in the soil for two or three weeks before becoming infective. When infective eggs are swallowed by man they hatch in the upper duodenum, the juveniles gradually developing

TABLE 10

Parasite	Definitive hosts	Location in hosts	Intermediate hosts	Pathogenic effects
Dirofilaria immitis	Dogs, cats, fur-bearers	Right ventricle, pulmonary artery	Mosquitoes	Cardiac, arterial and pulmonary lesions leading to dyspnoea, cough and tendency to tire easily
Dipetalonema spp.	Dogs	Peritoneal and pleural cavities	Midges (*Culicoides*), dog fleas, dog lice	Apparently slight
Parafilaria multipapillosa	Equines (in eastern countries)	Subcutaneous and intermuscular connective tissue	Unknown	Haemorrhagic subcutaneous nodules
P. bovicola	Cattle (in India)	Subcutaneous connective tissue	Unknown	Haemorrhagic subcutaneous nodules
Brugia spp.	Dogs, cats		See above	
*Onchocera gibsoni**	Cattle	Subcutaneous connective tissue of the hind limbs	Midges (*Culicoides*)	Fibrous subcutaneous nodules
Elaeophora poeli	Cattle	Lumen and wall of the aorta	Unknown	Nodules in aortic wall but no symptoms
Setaria equina	Equines	Peritoneal cavity	Unknown	Fibrinous peritonitis
S. cervi	Cattle	Peritoneal cavity	Stable-flies	None
S. digitata	Cattle,† sheep, goats, horses (man)	Peritoneal cavity (cattle), central nervous system and eye (other hosts)	Mosquitoes	Symptomless in normal hosts;† but causes epidemic cerebrospinal disease in sheep, goats and horses characterized by paralysis of limbs
S. congolensis	Pigs	Peritoneal cavity	Unknown	None
Neurofilaria cornellensis	Sheep (America)	Brain and spinal cord	Unknown	Inco-ordination of movement followed by paralysis
Suifilaria suis	Pigs (South Africa)	Subcutaneous and intermuscular connective tissue	Unknown	Vesicular skin eruptions, connective tissue nodules
Stephanofilaria spp.	Cattle	Skin	Unknown—blood-sucking arthropod?	Inflammatory pruritic skin lesions (verminous dermatitis or cascado)—Java, Sumatra, Celebes Hump sore—India

* Several other species of the genus *Onchocera* occur in the ligaments and tendons of cattle and equines and are transmitted by midges or black-flies; but none are seriously pathogenic.

† Cattle (including oxen and zebu) are the normal hosts of this species, which occurs in Ceylon, India, Burma, Japan and Korea. In Japan it commonly causes ocular filariasis of horses; and it has been suggested that it may transmit the virus of Japanese B. encephalitis to human beings and horses.

to maturity as they migrate slowly down the intestine towards the caecum. There are no reservoir hosts, although morphologically indistinguishable physiological races occur in monkeys and pigs. Man is not susceptible to infection with these forms. Light infections are symptomless. Heavy infections are characterised by abdominal pain, constipation or diarrhoea, vomiting, flatulence, anorexia, fever, loss of weight and neurotoxic symptoms (irritability, insomnia, giddiness). Very heavy infections also show dyspnoea, cardiac dilatation and anaemia; and may terminate fatally.

Trichinella spiralis **(the trichina worm).** This species, although essentially cosmopolitan in distribution, is commoner in Europe and the U.S.A. than elsewhere; and is rare or absent in Moslem countries. The adults are very small worms (1·5–5 mm by 40–60 microns) which live attached to or buried in the mucosa of the upper part of the small intestine. The males are evacuated in the faeces after copulation, but the viviparous females burrow deeper in the intestinal wall and give birth to numerous first-stage juveniles which enter blood or lymph capillaries and are carried through the right heart and lungs to the arterial circulation by which they are distributed to all parts of the body. The juveniles escape from the capillaries, but are able to develop further only in the voluntary muscles, where they grow into the infective stage and become enclosed in an ellipsoidal host cyst. If the infected muscle is eaten by another potential host the infective juveniles are liberated by digestion and rapidly develop to sexual maturity in the duodenum.

T. spiralis is normally a parasite of rats, the life-cycle being adapted to the cannibalistic habits of these rodents; but any mammal feeding on an infected rat is liable to become infected. Pigs are the most frequent alternative reservoir hosts. Man acquires the infection by consuming raw or under-cooked pork or pork products or bear meat. The great majority of infections are symptomless; but in severe cases, where the number of parasites is high, juveniles and adults burrowing in the intestinal wall may cause catarrhal enteritis with consequent abdominal pain, nausea and vomiting, diarrhoea, fever, and profuse perspiration. Juveniles migrating from the intestinal wall to the encystment sites may cause toxaemic effects, of which headache and oedema of the face and hands are the most pronounced. Invasion of the muscles by the juveniles is accompanied by interstitial myositis with resulting symptoms ranging from muscular tenderness to severe rheumatoid pains. Difficulty in breathing, mastication, swallowing and speech may follow heavy invasion of the muscles involved. In the final phase, the encystment period, which is reached one to two months after infection, there is either gradual abatement of symptoms followed by recovery, or the condition of the patient worsens until death supervenes, usually as a result of generalised toxaemia, secondary pneumonia or cardiac failure.

A number of species of Trichuroidea occur in domestic animals:

Trichuris ovis in the caecum of goats, sheep, cattle and other ruminants,
T. globulosa in the caecum of camels, sheep, goats, cattle and other ruminants,
T. vulpis in the intestine of dogs and foxes,
T. trichiura races in monkeys and pigs. (See above.)

Species of the related genus *Capillaria* occur in the intestine or the crop and oesophagus of fowls, pigeons, turkeys, ducks and other birds, and in the small intestine or urinary bladder and kidney pelvis of fur-bearing mammals. Many of them are stated to utilise earthworms as intermediate hosts.

Hepaticola hepaticola occurs in the liver of dogs, rabbits and many other mammals, including man.
Eucoleus aerophilus occurs in the trachea and bronchi of dogs, cats and fur-bearing mammals.

All of these veterinary forms are pathogenic to a greater or lesser degree. The species of *Trichuris* cause similar effects in animal hosts to those which they produce in man, especially in canine hosts. *Capillaria* infections in birds range from the completely symptomless to those showing loss of appetite, severe emaciation and anaemia, dyspnoea, inco-ordination and paralysis, with fatal termination. *Capillaria* infection in fur-bearers causes haemorrhagic enteritis, particularly in mink. *H. hepatica* produces hepatomegaly and liver dysfunction; while *E. aerophilus* is responsible for chronic tracheitis and bronchitis with resulting dyspnoea, anaemia and emaciation.

Higuerolatex and dithiazanine are the drugs of choice in the treatment of human whipworm infection. In animals, dithiazanine, diphenylamine and *n*-butyl chloride are effective. Intra-caecal infection of a mixture of the last-named drug together with hydrogen peroxide and nicotine is particularly efficient in removing the

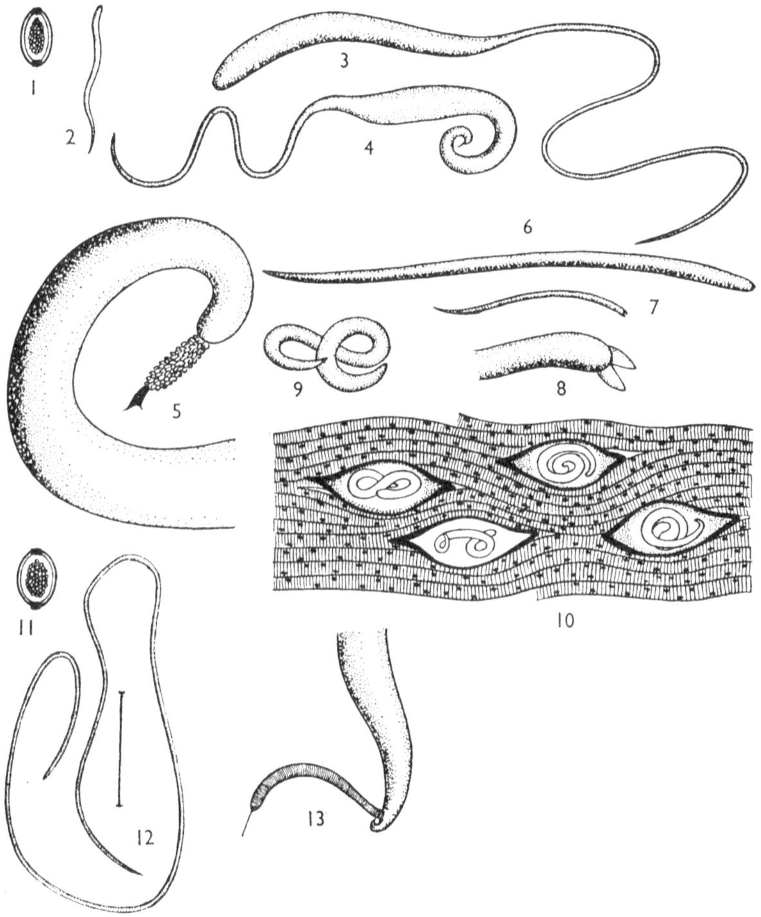

FIG. 19*a*. Whipworm and Trichina Worm

1 *Trichuris trichiura*—egg.
2 —first-stage juvenile.
3 —adult female worm.
4 —adult male worm.
5 —posterior end of male worm showing spicule sheath and spicule.
6 *Trichinella spiralis*—adult female worm.
7 —adult male worm.
8 —posterior end of male worm.
9 —juvenile.
10 —encysted juveniles in striated muscle.
11 *Capillaria columbae*—egg.
12 —posterior end of male worm.
13 —adult worm.

parasites. In cattle and sheep, butyl *n*-phenylthiocarbamate and 1 : 8 : dihydroxyanthraquinone have given good results. Piperazine is without effect.

Prevention of whipworm infection in man involves personal hygiene, sanitary disposal of faeces, prevention of promiscuous defaecation and avoidance of the use of unsterilised night-soil as fertiliser. In animals, cleanliness and pasture rotation alone are available as prophylactic measures.

It is generally accepted that no treatment is effective against *Trichinella spiralis* infection in man. In animals this is also the case, although promising results have been reported from the use of the two drugs methydrine (2-(β-methoxyethyl)-pyridine) administered subcutaneously and thiabendazole (2-(4′-thiazalyl-benzimidadzole) given by mouth in both whipworm and *T. spiralis* infection.

Prevention of trichinelliasis in man involves the elimination of the disease in pigs, by feeding only sterilised garbage and by strict anti-rodent campaigns; and the avoidance of transmission to man by meat inspection, and by the cooking or deep-freezing for long periods of all pork and pork products intended for human consumption.

Dioctophymoidea

A single species is an uncommon parasite of man.

Dioctophyme renale (**the giant kidney worm**). This very large (14–100 cm by 0·5–1 cm), red worm is essentially cosmopolitan in distribution, but occurs more frequently in Europe and North America than other parts of the world. The adults inhabit the abdominal cavity of the definitive host and invade the kidneys, whence the popular name. The eggs pass out in the urine and hatch if ingested by a suitable species of annelid worm. After undergoing development in the first intermediate host the juveniles encyst in the tissues of crayfish and only proceed further to the infective stage if the crayfish is eaten by a fresh-water fish. The definitive host acquires the infection by consuming infected fish raw or under-cooked. Dog, fur-bearers and other fish-eating mammals serve as reservoir hosts, human infection being relatively rare. Extensive destruction of kidney tissue results from this infection and local pain, sometimes excruciating, nervous symptoms, haematuria and uraemia are the typical sequelae.

A related but smaller (2–4 cm) form, *Hystrichis tricolor*, occurs in the proventricular glands of ducks, producing nodules and destroying the tissues. The life-cycle is unknown.

Surgery is the only possible treatment in cases of infection with the giant kidney worm; but infection is easily avoided by eating no raw or under-cooked fish, and by not feeding such fish to dogs.

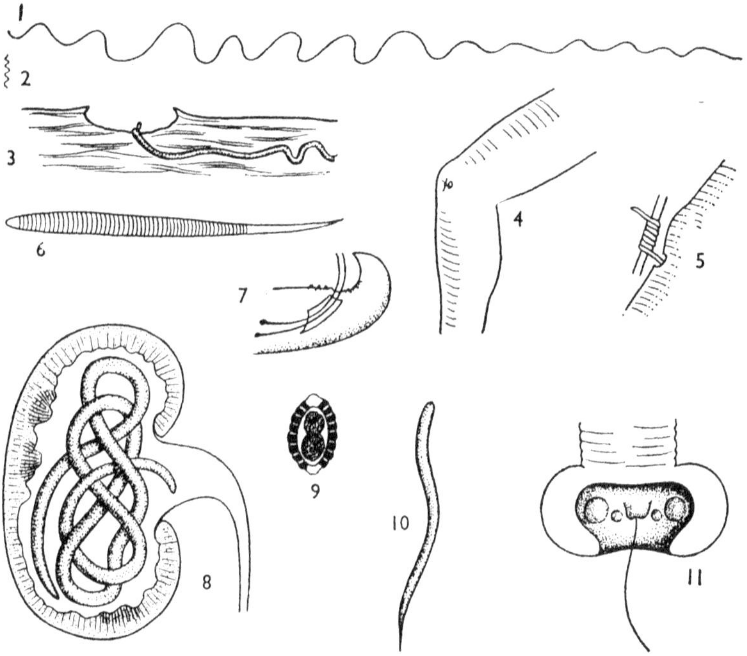

FIG. 20. Guinea Worm and Giant Kidney Worm

1 *Dracunculus medinensis*—adult female (one-fifth nat. size).
2 —adult male (one-fifth nat. size).
3 —section of ulcer showing female worm in subcutaneous tissues.
4 —ulcer on human knee with female worm partly withdrawn and rolled on a stick.
5 —enlarged view of female worm being withdrawn through ulcer by rolling on a stick.
6 —free-swimming first-stage larva.
7 —posterior end of male worm in side-view, showing spicules clasped by gubernacular sheath.
8 *Dioctophyme renale*—adult female worm coiled within a partly-destroyed kidney.
9 —egg.
10 —free-swimming first-stage larva.
11 —posterior end of male worm showing single spicule protruding from bursal cup.

HIRUDINEA
(LEECHES)

Medicinal Leeches

Hirudo medicinalis and several other species of Hirudinea have been extensively used in the past for the purpose of blood-letting. Indeed, until the latter half of the nineteenth century their employment was regarded almost as a panacea and special leech farms existed to supply the enormous demand by hospitals and private practitioners. The fact that many bloodliving pathogenic micro-organisms—protozoans, bacteria and viruses—can survive unharmed for several days in the gut of the leech, indicates that this animal must have been frequently the means of spreading infection. Leeches are still very occasionally used in the treatment of thrombosis, phlebitis, polycythaemia vera and hypertension unaccompanied by anaemia.

Pathogenic Leeches

A number of species of leech attack the external surface of the body of man and domestic animals, causing inconvenience, blood-loss, and sometimes more serious symptoms. Land-leeches belonging to the genera *Haemadipsa* and *Philaemon* are a serious menace in many parts of South and East Asia, some Pacific Islands, North Australia, Madagascar, and Central and South America. They are usually associated with tropical rain-forest and other forms of lush vegetation resulting from hot, damp conditions. They are very active, springing onto passing mammals from the leaves and boughs where they lie in wait. In the Mediterranean area an aquatic species belonging to the genus *Placobdella* occurs in springs and water-cress beds and attacks man and domestic animals. The bite of all these leeches is painless but the wound heals slowly and haemorrhage may be serious in cases of multiple attack. Any irritant, such as alcohol, brine or vinegar, will cause the animals to drop off and the wounds may then be bathed with an astringent, antiseptic solution. Prevention involves the choice between protective clothing and repellent ointments or paints containing dibutyl or dimethyl phthallate.

In many parts of the world aquatic leeches of the genus *Limnatis* sometimes gain entry to the upper parts of the digestive and respiratory tracts via the mouth or nostrils of persons bathing or washing in the waters of infested springs, brooks, ponds or lakes. They attach themselves to the mucous membrane, causing irritation, haemorrhage and considerable discomfort. In parts of India a particularly active species—*Dinobdella ferox*—attacks man and

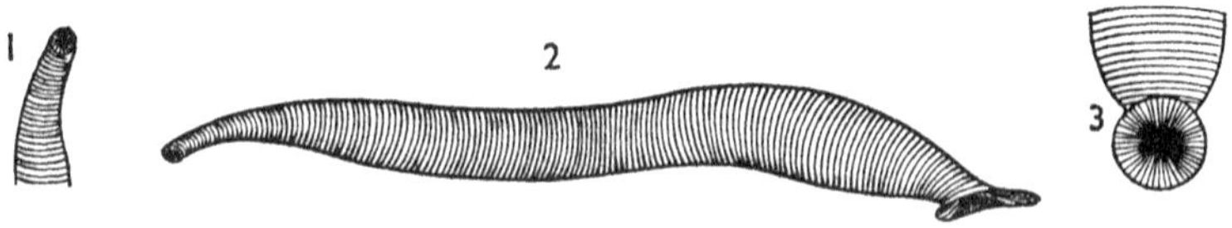

FIG. 21. Medicinal Leech (*Hirudo medicinalis*)

1 Ventral view of anterior end to show mouth and oral sucker.
2 Side view of entire animal.
3 Ventral view of posterior end to show posterior sucker.

animals in this way, looping rapidly up the arm or face to enter the mouth or nostrils. Treatment involves anaesthetizing the leech with cocaine and removing it with forceps.

All of these species can affect domestic animals. Species of *Limnatis* are particularly troublesome in certain areas, such as South-East Europe and West Africa. Horses are especially prone to the attacks of land leeches. Aquatic birds may be severely affected by small leeches belonging to the genera *Dina*, *Protoclepsis*, *Placobdella* and *Theromyzon*, which establish themselves in the nasal cavities.

CHAPTER 4

ENTOMOLOGY

NATURE AND CLASSIFICATION OF ARTHROPODA OF MEDICAL AND VETERINARY IMPORTANCE

Medical and veterinary entomology is generally taken to include the study of all members of the phylum Arthropoda which are important in connection with human or animal disease and discomfort; although in the strict sense of the word it should include only the study of insects. The arthropods are characterised by having a bilaterally symmetrical, metamerically segmented body; a chitinous exoskeleton; a well-developed head with eyes and antennae or pedipalps; paired, jointed appendages; a haemocoelic body-cavity; and a dorsal heart. The phylum is subdivided into the following classes:

(1) **Onychophora (Walking Worms)**

Soft-bodied terrestrial forms with unjointed legs.

(2) **Crustacea (Crabs, Lobsters, Shrimps, Water-fleas,** etc.)

Mainly aquatic forms, breathing by gills or through the skin and having variously modified biramous appendages including two pairs of antennae and paired natatory structures (swimmerets) on the underside of the abdomen.

(3) **Chilopoda (Centipedes)**

Elongate, flattened, carnivorous, terrestrial forms having one pair of legs to each segment and a pair of poison claws anteriorly. They breathe by tracheae.

(4) **Diplopoda (Millipedes)**

Elongate, cylindrical, herbivorous forms having the segments fused in pairs so that there appear to be two pairs of legs to each segment. They breathe by tracheae. Poison claws are lacking.

(5) **Insecta (Insects)**

Mainly terrestrial forms having the body sharply divided into head, thorax and abdomen; the head bears a pair of compound eyes and a pair of uniramous antennae; the thorax bears three pairs of walking legs and, in most orders, two pairs of wings. Breathing is by tracheae. This very large phylum is divided into many orders, of which the following are important in medical and veterinary science:

(*a*) ORTHOPTERA. This order includes forms with incomplete metamorphosis, leathery fore-wings and biting mouthparts, such as the cockroaches, grasshoppers, locusts and crickets.

(*b*) HEMIPTERA. The members of this order, which includes the bed-bugs and assassin-bugs, also have an incomplete metamorphosis, but the fore-wings are thick and leathery at the base only and the mouthparts form a jointed suctorial beak.

(*c*) ANOPLURA. These forms are known as the sucking lice. They are small, dorsoventrally flattened, wingless insects with sucking mouthparts. Metamorphosis is incomplete.

(*d*) MALLOPHAGA. This order includes the biting lice, which are also small, depressed, wingless forms with incomplete metamorphosis; but the mouthparts are adapted for biting.

(*e*) DIPTERA. This is a large and important order, the members of which are sometimes known as the two-winged flies. It includes the mosquitoes, midges and gnats, sand-flies, horse-flies, deer-flies, tsetse-flies, house-flies, stable-flies, horn-flies and bluebottles. Size varies from minute to large; metamorphosis is complete; one pair of wings only is present, the hinder pair having been modified into club-shaped balancers or halteres; and mouth-parts are of the piercing-sucking or sponging type.

(*f*) SIPHONAPTERA. This order of laterally compressed, wingless forms with complete metamorphosis, piercing-sucking mouthparts and long legs adapted for jumping, comprises the fleas and chiggers.

(*g*) HYMENOPTERA. This order includes the bees, wasps and ants. Size varies from minute to large; two pairs of inter-locking membranous wings are present; metamorphosis is complete; mouth-parts are of the biting or biting-lapping type; and in the female an ovipositor is present which may be adapted as a sting by means of which poison may be injected into prey or enemy.

Mouthparts in insects are basically of two types—the biting type and the sucking type. The former vary little; but the latter may be adapted for stabbing and piercing, as in the mosquito, or for scraping and sponging, as in the house-fly. In insects with incomplete metamorphosis the young stages are nymphs with compound eyes, in which the wings develop externally and the change into the adult form is gradual. In insects with complete metamorphosis, on the other hand, the young stages are larvae in which compound eyes are lacking, the wings develop internally, and the change into the adult form is abrupt.

(6) **Arachnoidea**

These are mainly terrestrial forms having the body divided into cephalothorax and abdomen. The cephalothorax bears four pairs of walking legs, a pair of usually sensory pedipalps, and a pair of biting chelicerae. Three orders only are of importance in medical and veterinary science:

(*a*) ARANEIDA. This very large order comprises the spiders, in which the abdomen is unsegmented; the chelicerae are provided with poison glands and ducts; and breathing is carried out by means of lung-books. Size varies greatly.

(*b*) SCORPIONIDA. This order comprises the scorpions, which are viviparous forms having a long segmented abdomen, slender posteriorly and carrying a sting at the end. The pedipalps are large and modified as chelate claws for seizing and grasping. Most species are large.

(*c*) ACARINA. The members of this order—the mites and ticks—are mainly very small forms in which the body is neither clearly segmented nor divided into cephalothorax and abdomen. Many are almost globular in form. Breathing is by tracheae. In many species the chelicerae and pedipalps are modified to form sucking and piercing mouthparts.

(7) **Xiphosura**

These are aquatic forms closely related to the Arachnoidea and known popularly as king crabs. They are of no medical or veterinary importance.

(8) **Pentastomida**

This exclusively parasitic group have received the popular name of tongue-worms. They have an elongate, tongue-like body, cylindrical or moniliform, showing pseudosegmentation but no main subdivisions. The mouth is provided with two pairs of hollow, retractile, claw-like jaws. The life-cycle involves an intermediate host and both young stages and mature forms are endoparasitic in vertebrate hosts.

Arthropods are of medical and veterinary importance in the following ways:

(1) As **biological vectors** or **intermediate hosts,** i.e. forms in which a parasite undergoes an obligatory phase of development before being transmitted to the definitive host. Thus, certain species of mosquitoes are obligatory intermediate hosts of the malaria parasites which they transmit.
(2) As **mechanical vectors,** i.e. forms by which a parasite is mechanically transmitted from one host to another without undergoing any development during the process. Thus house-flies transmit cysts of *Entamoeba histolytica* on their feet and in their vomit-drops and faeces.
(3) As **pathogens,** i.e. forms which actually cause disease; such as certain species of Diptera which cause the condition known as myiasis and the mites which cause scabies and mange.
(4) As **venomous biters** and **stingers;** such as, for example, the scorpions, certain species of spiders, and many bees, wasps and ants.
(5) As **irritating ectoparasites;** such as the fleas, mosquitoes, gnats and midges, sand-flies, black-flies, deer-flies, horse-flies, lice, bed-bugs and assassin-bugs. Many of these forms are also mechanical or biological vectors.

MOSQUITOES
(CULICIDAE)

Distribution and Morphology

The members of the dipterous family Culicidae are the most important group of insects from the medical and veterinary point of view. They are small, cosmopolitan flies which occur in abundance from the polar regions to the equator. The body, especially the abdomen, is slender; the long, narrow wings have one or more cross-veins at or beyond the middle, lack an extra seventh vein, and show flat scales around the posterior margin and along the longitudinal veins; the head carries a long proboscis adapted, in the females of many species, for sucking blood; and the antennae are generally plumose in the males and thread-like in the females.

Life-cycle and Habits

The eggs are usually laid on the surface of water, either singly, or in groups, or in raft-shaped masses. Hatching depends on temperature and normally occurs in two to three days; but in some species eggs remain dormant through the winter or during drought.

The active, wriggling larvae are aquatic, living submerged in the water of wells, ditches, streams, pools, lakes and swamps, but coming to the surface to breathe air through special openings (respiratory siphons) in the eighth abdominal segment. They have biting mouthparts with complex brush-like structures in constant motion, wafting food particles, such as minute organisms and fragments of organic matter floating in the water, into the mouth. There is a large head, a thorax consisting of three fused segments, and a long abdomen of nine segments, the last of which carries four finger-like tracheal gills. The larval stage lasts from six days to several weeks, depending on the temperature and food-supply; but ten days is a normal average span. During this period the larva moults four times, the last moult producing the next, or pupal, stage.

The pupa, is also aquatic but, although free and active, it does not feed. It comes to the surface to breathe air through two trumpet-like tubes on the thorax. The body is bent in the shape of a question-mark. The head and thorax are enclosed in a transparent shell or case through which the developing compound eyes, legs and wings can be seen. The last abdominal segment carries a pair of paddles. This stage also lasts for a variable time, but four or five days is usual.

The adult or imago emerges from the pupa when the latter rises to the surface for the last time and the pupal skin splits dorsally. The adult rests on the floating pupal skin for a while to dry its wings; and then flies away. The life-span ranges from four days to just over a month, depending on species, food and environmental conditions; but some species can hibernate over the winter. Mosquitoes do not fly high and do not range actively more than two or three kilometres from the breeding place; but they may be carried long distances by the wind. Most species are nocturnal in habit, being especially active at twilight. They are attracted by warmth, light and animals. Mating occurs during flight. The females of most species require a blood-meal in order to produce fertile eggs. Several generations may be produced annually in warm climates.

Habitats vary, some species being essentially jungle and forest dwellers, others are rural, and yet others are urban or domestic forms.

Medical and Veterinary Importance

The importance of mosquitoes to man depends primarily upon their ability to transmit various diseases of man and domestic animals, the most serious of which are as follows:

(1) **Malaria.** Human malaria is transmitted only by members of the genus *Anopheles*. About one hundred species of this genus have been incriminated in various parts of the world, the majority being of local importance only. The major vectors which are of wide distribution are listed in Table 11.

(2) **Yellow fever.** This frequently fatal virus infection characterised by necrosis of the liver and kidney, high fever and black vomit, was a widespread scourge in Europe, the U.S.A., Central and Southern America and Africa, before the discovery of the vector. It effectively prevented the building of the Panama Canal and it was this fact which stimulated the research which eventually led to its conquest. It exists in two forms—an endemic jungle form in reservoir hosts (mainly monkeys) transmitted by various species of wild mosquitoes, and an epidemic urban form transmitted by the domestic mosquito *Aedes aegypti*, which breeds in any receptacle holding water in and around human habitations. Effective control measures and quarantine regulations have eliminated the urban disease, but men entering the endemic jungle areas may become infected and carry the disease back to urban areas, where it will spread if *A. aegypti* is present.

(3) **Dengue.** This tropical virus infection characterised by skin eruption and severe muscular pains is also transmitted by *Aedes aegypti*, except in South-Eastern and Eastern Asia where the vector is *A. albopictus*. The latter species breeds near dwellings in water trapped in bamboo stems.

(4) **Filariasis.** *Wuchereria bancrofti* is transmitted in nature by at least twelve species of *Culex*, six species of *Aedes*, twenty-five species of *Anopheles* and seven species of *Mansonia*. The most important of these vectors are shown in Table 12.

Brugia malayi is transmitted in nature by at least seven species of *Mansonia* (especially *M. annulifera* in India) and two species of *Anopheles*.

(5) **Encephalitis.** Various diseases of this type are transmitted by

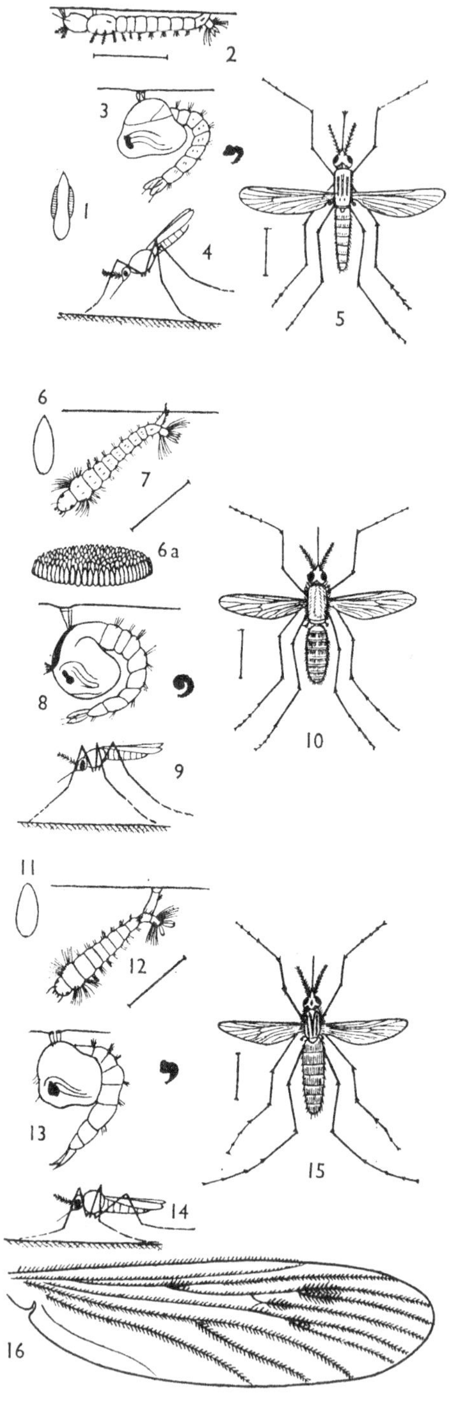
1
2
3
4
5
6
6a
7
8
9
10
11
12
13
14
15
16

TABLE 11

Species	Distribution	Breeding places	Remarks
Anopheles maculipennis	Cosmopolitan	Any fresh or brackish water	Many subspecies and races which vary in their importance as vectors
A. gambiae	Africa, Madagascar, Mauritius, Introduced into Brazil in 1930 and eradicated in 1939	Any stagnant water exposed to the sun, especially grassy pools and streams	Probably the most potent vector owing to the domesticated habits of the adults
A. funestus	Africa	Shady, grass-edged, sluggish streams with clean water	Adapted to lower temperatures and higher altitudes than *A. gambiae*
A. subpictus *A. vagus*	India	Puddles, ponds and rice-fields	
A. culifacies	Southern Asia (especially India) and Arabia	Clear, sunny pools and irrigation channels	
A. quadrimaculatus	U.S.A.	Clean, still, sunny water, covered with surface vegetation	Principal vector in the southern U.S.A.
A. punctipennis	U.S.A.	Cool shady pools	
A. pseudopunctipennis	Central and Southern America	Clear, sunlit pools; especially receding streams	Important vector in Mexico and South America
A. punctulatus	Australia, South Pacific, Indonesia	Stagnant swamps; shady forest pools; rice-fields; temporary puddles	

FIG. 22. Mosquitoes

1 *Anopheles* sp.—egg.
2 —larva.
3 —pupa.
4 —resting position of adult.
5 —adult female (dorsal view).
6 *Culex* sp.—single egg.
6a —egg-raft.
7 —larva.
8 —pupa.
9 —resting position of adult.
10 —adult female (dorsal view).
11 *Aedes* sp.—egg.
12 —larva.
13 —pupa.
14 —resting position of adult.
15 —adult female (dorsal view).
16 Generalised view of mosquito wing.

TABLE 12

Species	Distribution	Breeding places	Remarks
Culex fatigans (syn. *C. quinquifasciatus*)	Tropics and subtropics	Any collection of still water, e.g. tubs and storage tanks, near human dwellings	Also transmits *Dirofilaria immitis* of dogs. Nocturnal
C. pipiens	U.S.A., Europe, China and parts of South America	Polluted fresh-water—very slowly moving or stagnant	Common house mosquitoes. Main vector in Egypt and China. Nocturnal
Aedes aegypti	Tropics and subtropics (urban)	Collections of water in tree-holes and receptacles, tanks, tubs, etc., in the immediate vicinity of human habitations	Nocturnal
A. scutellaris	Pacific area	Small collections of water containing decayed organic matter, e.g. coconut shells, holes in trees, empty tins and bottles lying about	Readily enters houses—but is not a domestic species. Diurnal
Anopheles darlingi	South America	Pools and puddles beside rivers and roads	
A. gambiae	See Table of Malaria Vectors above		
A. punctulatus	See Table of Malaria Vectors above		

species of *Culex* and *Aedes*, especially *C. pipiens*, *C. tarsalis*, *C. taeniorhynchus* and *A. aegypti*.

(6) **Myiasis.** Infection with the tropical bot-fly *Dermatobia hominis* is transmitted mechanically by *Psorophora lutzi*, *P. ferox* and *P. cyanescens*. The female *D. hominis* cements her eggs to the abdomen of the mosquito, and the warmth of the human body causes them to hatch when the mosquito feeds on man.

(7) **Yaws.** This venereal infection can be transmitted mechanically by *Aedes aegypti* in South America.

(8) **Tularaemia.** Infection with *Pasteurella tularensis* may be mechanically transmitted by mosquitoes, especially in Norway, where the disease is widespread.

(9) **Mosquito dermatitis.** Some persons suffer severely from a form of allergic skin irritation caused by the bites of mosquitoes.

Control

Before control of mosquitoes is undertaken it is essential that the species involved should be identified and their breeding and other habits investigated in relation to human, climatic and topographic factors; so that rational and effective measures may be devised. The co-operation of the human populations involved is usually necessary if control measures are to be successful. The methods generally used are summarised below.

Measures directed against the larvae

(*a*) ALTERATION OF ENVIRONMENTAL CONDITIONS TO PREVENT BREEDING

(i) Draining or filling-in of all larger collections of stagnant water, such as pools, ponds and swamps.
(ii) Clearing vegetation along banks of streams and near dwellings.
(iii) Covering or removal of cisterns, wells and accidental or ornamental collections of water, including such objects as empty coconut shells and old bottles and tins, which may fill with water and become temporary breeding places.
(iv) Development of shade if larvae need sunshine; and vice versa.
(v) Frequent alterations of water level.
(vi) Increased rate of water flow.
(vii) Stream channelisation.

(*b*) USE OF LARVICIDAL CHEMICALS

(i) Certain oil mixtures form a film over the surface of the water which is not only toxic to the larvae on contact but also prevents them from breathing, so that they die of suffocation. Kerosene and diesel oil make an effective and toxic mixture. Oiling cannot be used if there is excessive vegetation, heavy rain or high evaporation.
(ii) Paris Green, distributed over the water as a fine dust, suitably diluted, is effective as a stomach poison (i.e. a poison which is toxic when ingested).
(iii) Pyrethrum, gammexane and DDT, dispersed as emulsions, fine dusts, aqueous suspensions or oil solutions, distributed by hand- or power-sprays or from aircraft, have proved effective.

(*c*) INTRODUCTION OF ENEMIES. Several species of small fish feed voraciously on mosquito larvae, e.g. *Gambusia affinis holbrooki* (warm countries only), *Aplocheilus panchax* (India) and *Leucaspius delineatus* (Ukraine).

Measures directed against the adults

(*a*) INSECTICIDAL SPRAYS. Pyrethrum, DDT and gammexane are used in various formulations either for immediate or for residual effect, both inside buildings and in the outdoor habitats of the mosquitoes. Resistant strains have developed to some of these insecticides.

(*b*) SCREENING. Bronze wire screening or cloth netting with eighteen meshes to the inch effectively prevents the ingress of mosquitoes if securely fixed over doors and windows.

(*c*) ANIMAL BARRIERS. Domestic animals stationed between the breeding grounds of the mosquitoes and human habitations divert a large proportion of the adults in the case of zoophilous species.

(*d*) REPELLENTS. Various substances, such as dibutyl phthallate, dimethyl phthallate, indalone, Rutger's 612, benzyl benzoate, and oils of cassia and citronella, are distasteful to mosquitoes and can be applied to the skin of the exposed parts of the body and to the clothing.

(*e*) PROTECTIVE CLOTHING. Head-nets, gloves, high boots and complete clothing give protection against mosquito bites provided that the material is of close enough weave. They are, however, uncomfortable and inconvenient to wear, especially in hot climates.

(*f*) TRAPS. Various types of traps have been used with some success to reduce the numbers of adult mosquitoes in limited areas. Space does not permit any consideration of these devices.

OTHER BLOOD-SUCKING FLIES

The following families of Diptera have representatives which are of medical and veterinary importance, chiefly on account of their blood-sucking habits and ability to transmit disease:

Psychodidae (Sand-flies; Moth-flies)

These are very small (1–3 mm), hairy, velvety-winged flies with short legs and short, broad bodies. They are weak fliers but active jumpers. The wings are broad and oval, evenly divided by ten, straight, parallel, longitudinal veins; and show few closed cells. The venation is obscured by hairs. The larvae live in water or damp, dark places, especially sewers or drains, and feed on algae, micro-organisms and decaying organic matter. Various species of the widely distributed genus *Phlebotomus* transmit sand-fly fever, oriental sore, kala-azar, espundia and also bartonellosis (Oroya fever). Sand-flies are nocturnal in habit and have an irritating bite; are voracious blood-suckers; and are especially active at dusk and dawn. They rarely fly far from their breeding places or rise high above the ground, hence the incidence of *Phlebotomus*-transmitted diseases is always greatest among those living on the ground floor.

Ceratopogonidae (Midges and Gnats)

These are also very small (1–3 mm) flies. Swarms of them may often be seen in warm weather, dancing in the air over swamps and marshy places. The antennae are hairy; but the wings are bare or hairy at the margin only. The anterior wing veins are thicker than those behind; there are few closed cells; and the costal vein does not, as in mosquitoes, continue round to the posterior margin. The eggs are laid in water or on moist decaying organic matter; the larvae are aquatic, and the pupae are active. Few genera suck blood, but those which do bite man viciously, usually at dusk or by night. Members of the genus *Culicoides* transmit the filarial worms *Acanthocheilonema perstans* (*C. austeni*, *C. grahami*) and *Mansonella ozzardi* (*C. furens*) among human parasites. Other members of the same genus transmit *Dipetalonema* infection of dogs, *Onchocerca* infection of horses and other domestic livestock, *Haemoproteus* infection of ducks in America and blue-tongue of sheep in South Africa.

Simuliidae (Black-flies; Buffalo-gnats)

Small (1–5 mm), stoutly-built, dark-coloured, cosmopolitan flies with short, broad iridescent wings having stout anterior and weak posterior veins with no closed cells. The antennae are short and horn-like, and the large head is set low against the arched thorax, giving the fly a hump-backed appearance. Black-flies are abundant from the tropics to the sub-arctic in spring and early summer, especially near fast-running water.

The egg-masses are fastened by the females to the surface of stones, sticks and vegetation just below the surface of running waters. On hatching, the cylindrical larvae cling by means of a terminal hooked disc to the rocks and stones near which they find themselves, or to the carapace of fresh-water crabs. They frequent the swiftest parts of the streams, feeding on organic particles and micro-organisms by means of fan-shaped mouth-brushes, and breathing through short, retractile, anal gill-filaments. The pupae have thoracic tracheal gills and are encased in vase-shaped cocoons attached to submerged rocks and water-plants. The adults emerge under water, float to the surface in a bubble of air, and are on the wing before the current can drown them.

Both sexes are vicious, painful biters and blood-suckers, and their bites leave sore, itching, ulcerous lesions. Swarms of these flies cause great harm to cattle and other domestic stock, preventing them from grazing, provoking them to stampede and injure themselves, and even making them anaemic. Their attacks can be fatal. Species of the genus *Simulium* transmit human infection with the filarial worm *Onchocerca volvulus* (*S. damnosum* and *S. neavei* in Africa, *S. avidum*, *S. ochraceum* and *S. mooseri* in Central America). Other species of this genus transmit *Leucocytozoon* and *Haemoproteus* infections of various domestic birds and *Onchocerca* infection of cattle.

Tabanidae (Horse-flies; Deer-flies; Clegs)

These are large (10–25 mm), robust, cosmopolitan flies with a smooth, compact body, strong legs, and a short, broad head the upper part of which is almost entirely covered by the brilliant, iridescent eyes. The antennae are short and stiff with three dissimilar joints, and the short, thick, piercing-sucking mouthparts are provided with a fleshy labella for scraping and sponging as well. The wing venation is heavy and complex, with many closed cells; and the costal vein encircles the entire wing margin.

The females are blood-suckers, attacking any warm-blooded animals; but the males feed only on nectar and plant juices. Tabanids are active in hot, clear weather, are most frequent near water, and are strong fliers, easily able to keep up with a galloping horse. The bite is large and painful, but has no serious after-effects. The eggs are laid in batches near water, either in moist earth or leaf-mould or on the leaves and stems of water plants projecting above the surface. The slender, cylindrical larvae tunnel through moist soil or lead an aquatic existence, feeding on other small animals. The pupa stage is a chrysalis, from which the adult emerges through a dorsal slit.

Two species of the deer-fly *Chrysops* are important vectors of the filarial parasite *Loa loa* in West Africa (*C. silacea* and *C. dimidiata*) while a third species (*C. discalis*) transmits tularaemia in North and Central America. Various species of tabanid flies act as mechanical or biological vectors of trypanosomes parasitic in domestic animals; and many species also act as mechanical vectors of bacterial infections, such as anthrax, and virus infections, such as infectious anaemia of horses. Species of the genus *Tabanus* are vicious biters of man.

Muscidae (House-flies; Stable-flies; Horn-flies; and their Allies)

These are medium-sized (5–12 mm), cosmopolitan flies having a short, compact body which is usually greyish, black, or metallic blue or green in colour. The short, three-jointed antennae bear a plumose bristle (arista); and the eyes are large, touching at the top of the head in the males but separated there in the females. The mouthparts vary, being usually of the sponging and scraping type with a large labella; but some forms have piercing-sucking mouthparts and suck blood. The ample wings have complex venation with many closed cells. The eggs are laid in organic refuse or wounds, the whitish, elongate-conical larvae or 'gentles' feeding on the decaying organic matter or putrefying tissue, as the case may be. The oval, brownish pupae occur in drier places and often overwinter in cold climates. The adult emerges through a circular opening at the head end.

Both sexes of the stable-fly *Stomoxys calcitrans* and the horn-fly *Haematobia irritans* are vicious biters of man and domestic animals and, although not known to be vectors in nature, are able to transmit experimentally a number of human infections including poliomyelitis, tetanus, anthrax, trypanosomiasis and oriental sore. The irritation which they cause to domestic animals when present in large numbers results in loss of weight and condition and decreased milk yields. Stable-flies act as mechanical vectors of certain diseases of domestic stock, such as surra, anthrax and infectious anaemia of horses, and as biological vectors of others, such as infection with the nematode parasites *Habronema* and *Setaria*.

Glossinidae (Tsetse-flies)

The members of this tropical African family are superficially similar to the Muscidae, but are brownish in colour and have a long piercing-sucking proboscis extending in front of the head and enclosed by the palps. The long, clear to brownish wings overlap on the back when at rest, and differ in the details of their venation, the fourth longitudinal vein being curved sharply forward to meet a short transverse vein. Tsetse-flies are viviparous, the larvae maturing one at a time in the abdomen of the mother, nourished by the secretion of branched glands with teat-like openings near the inner end of the uterus. After birth the larva burrows into loose soil or sand, or conceals itself under dead leaves or other vegetable debris, and becomes a hard, dark-brown pupa, from which the adult emerges after three to four weeks. The adult lives from three to six months and produces up to twelve larvae during this period, which she deposits singly, at intervals of about eight days, in shady places where cover for the pupating young is available. Adult tsetse-flies require a high humidity and a mean annual temperature of not less than 21° C. They are strong fliers and cover considerable distances on the wing. Species of the genus *Glossina* spread trypanosomiasis of man and domestic animals (see Table 1). The three most important species affecting man are *G. palpalis*, *G. tachinoides* and *G. morsitans*. Several other species are local vectors of human trypanosomes or transmit animal trypanosomes only.

Hippoboscidae

The members of this aberrant family of Diptera are related to the Muscidae but show marked adaptation to existence as blood-sucking ectoparasites of mammals and birds. The body is dorso-ventrally flattened, the antennae reduced, the wings often lacking, the segmentation of the abdomen indistinct, and the terminal joints of the tarsi provided with special claws for clinging to the feathers or hairs of the host. Like the Glossinidae, the females are viviparous and give birth to larva which are ready to pupate. None are of medical importance but several are of veterinary importance:

(*a*) *Hippobosca* spp. These reddish flies with yellow spots attack horses, cattle, birds and dogs in warm countries. The female deposits single pupae in dry plant debris or soil in sheltered places. They attach themselves principally to the perineal and pubic skin, causing great irritation to the host, and also serving as biological vectors of *Trypanosoma theileri* and *Haemoproteus* spp. and as mechanical vectors of anthrax.

(*b*) *Melophagus ovinus* (**the sheep ked**). This cosmopolitan wingless brown form attacks sheep in all parts of the world. The larvae are attached by the female to the wool of the host and pupate

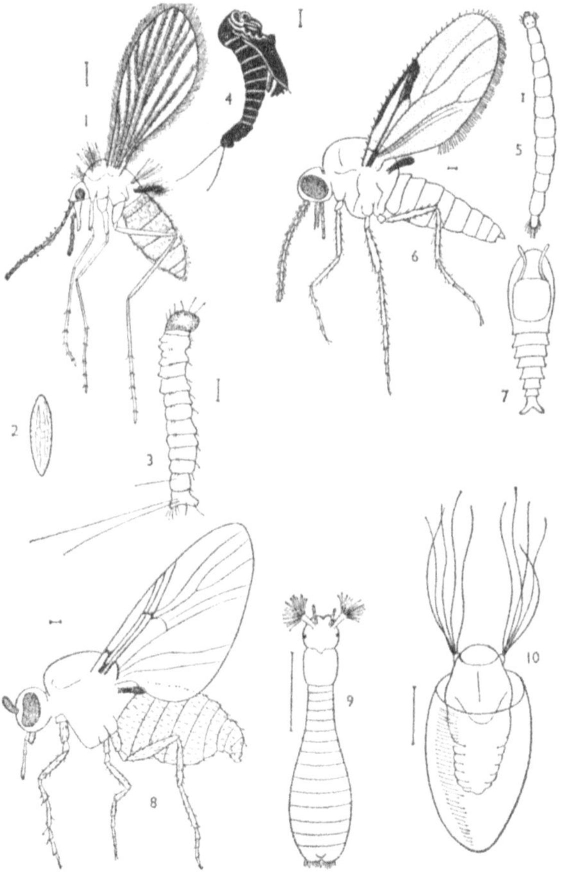

FIG. 23. Other Blood-sucking Flies

1 *Phlebotomus papatasii*—adult fly.
2 —egg.
3 —larva.
4 —pupa.
5 *Culicoides austeni*—larva.
6 —adult fly.
7 —pupa.
8 *Simulium damnosum*—adult fly.
9 —larva.
10 —pupa.

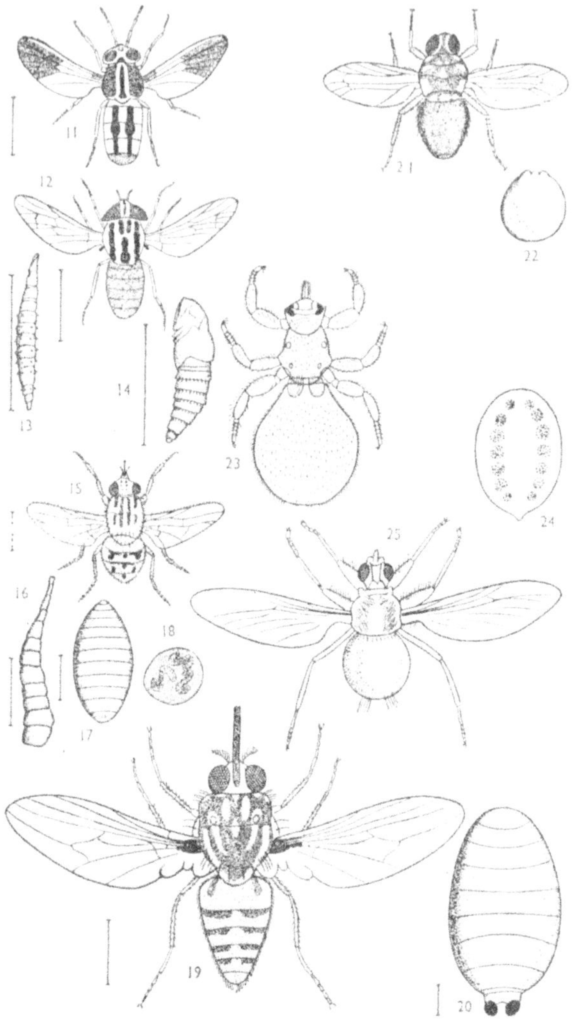

FIG. 23 (continued)

11 *Chrysops dimidiata*—adult fly.
12 *Tabanus* sp.—adult fly.
13 —larva.
14 —pupa.
15 *Stomoxys calcitrans*—adult fly.
16 —larva.
17 —puparium.
18 —posterior spiracle of larva.
19 *Glossina morsitans*—adult fly.
20 —puparium.
21 *Hippobosca rufipes*—adult fly.
22 —pupa.
23 *Melophagus ovinus*—adult fly.
24 —pupa.
25 *Pseudolynchia canariensis*—adult fly.

there. Heavy infections produce intense irritation and the resulting rubbing and scratching by the sheep damages the wool. The condition of the sheep deteriorate and in very severe cases even anaemia may result.

(*c*) *Pseudolynchia canariensis*. This dark brown fly attacks pigeons in warm countries, causing painful lesions and transmitting *Haemoproteus* infections.

Control

The control of sand-flies and midges resembles that of mosquitoes, but in the case of screens and nets a finer mesh is necessary on account of their smaller size, which enables them to slip easily through the meshes of mosquito netting. Breeding-places should be eliminated or treated with insecticides.

The control of black-flies is difficult because they are strong fliers and bite exclusively outdoors. Fly-proof clothes are the only effective protection. Larvae are killed by introducing insecticides such as gammexane and DDT into the water upstream from the breeding places, or by eliminating the fresh-water crabs to which some species attach themselves.

Protective clothing also provides the only effective protection against the bites of clegs and stable-flies, since they bite almost exclusively outdoors. Larval control involves elimination of breeding places, or their treatment with insecticides.

In the case of tsetse-flies control involves alteration of the habitat by bush clearance, to render it unsuitable for breeding; eradication of intermediate hosts, such as wild game animals in the case of *G. morsitans*; and the use of traps and hand-catching techniques for the adult flies. Bush clearance may consist of either eradicative clearing or protective clearing. The former aims to eradicate the tsetse-flies completely over a large area by completely removing the fly-belt vegetation of all primary breeding foci. The latter aims to reduce contact between fly and man by removing all fly-belt vegetation for at least one hundred metres around human habitations and places frequented by man, such as water-holes and road-river crossings. It is useless against *G. morsitans*. Eradicative clearing is more effective but more costly. Before clearing is undertaken the botany of the fly-belts and the exact habits and habitat of the species of *Glossina* involved must be carefully studied, since in some cases the fly can be exterminated by removal of only a few species of trees. Spraying or dusting of large areas of fly-infested country with suitable insecticide formulations from aeroplanes has had considerable success in recent years.

Except against sand-flies and midges, the use of repellents applied to the exposed areas of skin has not been successful.

The control of sheep keds and other hippoboscids is a special problem, since the whole life-cycle is passed on the host. Shearing, and dipping, using gammexane or DDT formulations, are most effective; but power-spraying with chordane or toxaphene is also employed.

NON-BLOODSUCKING FLIES

A number of dipterous species which do not suck blood or bite man or domestic animals are yet of great medical and veterinary importance, either because they are mechanical vectors of disease-causing organisms or because they have parasitic larvae and themselves produce disease. The former are known as filth-flies, the latter as myiasis-producers. Six families are involved.

Muscidae (House-flies)

The morphological characteristics and life-cycle of the members of this family have already been given above. The most important non-blood-sucking species is **the common house-fly,** *Musca demestica*. This medium-sized (8 mm), dark grey insect with the four characteristic longitudinal black stripes on the dorsum of the thorax has scraping-sponging mouthparts with a prominent labella. The adults live for about a month; and since the whole life-cycle from egg to adult can be completed in little over a week in hot weather, vast numbers of this pest may occur during the hot season in temperate climates and all the year round in tropical climates, unless effective control measures are undertaken. On account of their habit of passing from faeces to human food carrying filth on their feet, of regurgitating a vomit-drop before feeding, and of defaecation in the act of ingestion, house-flies regularly act as mechanical vectors of the following pathogens:

Salmonella spp. (typhoid and paratyphoid fevers);
Shigella spp. (bacterial dysentery);
Vibrio cholerae (cholera);
Entamoeba histolytica (amoebic dysentery) and other intestinal Protozoa;

Ascaris lumbricoides and other intestinal nematodes;
Poliomyelitis virus;
Trachoma virus;
Mycobacterium tuberculosis (tuberculosis);
Pasteurella pestis (bubonic plague);
Pasteurella tularensis (tularaemia);
Bacillus anthracis (anthrax);
Brucella spp. (Malta fever, undulant fevers, abortion in cows);
Treponema pertenue (yaws).

They can even spread leishmaniasis and trypanosomiasis by licking the blood drops from interrupted vector feeds.

Anthomyidae

The members of this family are in general similar to the Muscidae but are smaller and narrower and differ in the details of their wing venation. The larvae occur in decaying vegetable matter, stale faeces and the like. The habits, and therefore the medical and veterinary importance, of the adults are the same as those of *Musca domestica.* The two most important species are **the lesser house-fly,** *Fannia canicularis,* and **the latrine fly,** *F. scalaris.*

Calliphoridae (Blow-flies)

The members of this family also closely resemble the Muscidae, in which some authors include them as a sub-family. There are slight but constant differences in the hairs, antennae and wings. Most have a metallic sheen. Some species produce myiasis while others are typical filth flies. The most important are:

(*a*) *Chrysomyia bezziana* (**the Old World screw-worm fly**). This is a metallic blue fly with a bright green thorax, four black stripes on the prescutum, and an orange face. It lays its eggs on the skin of man and domestic animals, and in wounds, the larvae feeding principally on diseased tissue.

Several other species of this genus are sheep blow-flies, and lay their eggs on the skin and wool of these animals, the larvae having similar habits to those of *C. bezziana.*

(*b*) *Callitroga americana* (*Cochliomyia hominovorax*) (**the American screw-worm fly**). This is another bluish-green fly with a metallic sheen and an orange face; but the prescutum carries only three longitudinal black stripes. The eggs are laid on unbroken skin or mucous membrane, or in wounds. The larvae, which have a screwlike appearance owing to the spiral arrangement of their spines, bore into the tissues, destroying even cartilage and bone. If located in the nose or ear they may penetrate the brain and cause death. The adults are very strong fliers and travel long distances. A related species—*C. macellaria*—is similar in distribution, habits and appearance.

(*c*) *Cordylobia anthropophaga* (**the Tumbu fly**). This Central African species is a yellowish-grey insect with black spots on the abdomen and brown wings. It is an obligatory feeder on living flesh. The eggs are laid on the ground or in clothing contaminated with urine or sweat. The larvae penetrate the skin when activated by the warmth of the body and develop in the subcutaneous tissue, forming a painful boil-like lesion from which they emerge to pupate on the ground. It parasitises dogs, rabbits and other domestic animals, as well as man.

(*d*) *Auchmeromyia luteola*. This is another tropical African form which is apparently specific to man. It is a brownish fly that frequents native huts and lays its eggs in crevices of the floor, especially where urine has been voided. The larvae, known as **Congo floor maggots,** climb onto human beings while they are asleep and suck blood, dropping off when fully fed. This usually occurs at night. During the day they shelter in cracks in the floor. Pupation also takes place in this situation.

(*e*) *Calliphora* spp. (**bluebottles**). This cosmopolitan genus includes species which are typical filth flies, laying their eggs in animal refuse and carcasses and resembling house-flies in appearance and habits. They are, however, larger and have blue metallic bodies. Such are *C. vomitoria* and *C. erythrocephala*. But it also includes several species such as *C. stygia* which are typical myiasis-producers, laying their eggs in wounds or on the soiled wool of sheep. These forms are principally of importance in Australia; but *C. erythrocephala* and *C. vomitoria* have both been incriminated in the United Kingdom.

(*f*) *Lucilia* spp. (**greenbottles**). The members of this genus are also typically filth-flies, the eggs being laid and the larvae developing in organic refuse and faeces, carcasses of animals and the like. The adults generally have metallic coppery-green bodies. Certain species are, however, very important in the larval stage as myiasis-producers. *L. caesar*, a European form, and *L. serenissima*, **the bazaar-fly** of South India, can both produce this condition in man. *L. cuprina* and *L. sericata* are the most important producers of blow-fly strike in sheep, the former in Australia and South Africa, and the latter in the United Kingdom.

(*g*) *Phormia* spp. (**blackbottles**). These forms are similar to the two preceding genera but the adults have black metallic bodies. *P. regina* causes blow-fly strike of sheep in Canada and the United States of America, while *P. terrae-novae* has been incriminated in this country.

(*h*) *Booponus intonsus* (**the foot-maggot fly**). This light yellow fly lays its eggs on the coronet and pastern of goats and cattle in Celebes and the Philippine Islands, the larvae causing lameness.

Despite the fact that some of these flies affect man, it is as a cause of blow-fly strike (myiasis) of sheep that they are of chief importance to man. Large, irritating or painful inflamed lesions are formed, especially in the breech and around the tail, and the surrounding wool becomes moist, discoloured and evil-smelling. The animals cease to feed, and malnutrition may lead to death in severe cases.

Sarcophagidae (Flesh-flies)

These are large (10–14 mm) flies with conspicuous white stripes on the thorax and spots on the abdomen. They resemble the Muscidae except for slight differences in the wing venation and antennae and the fact that the abdomen is longer and narrower. The larvae of some species are parasitic in other insects while the larvae of others develop in dung, garbage, the carcasses of dead animals, wounds, or the nasal passages and stomach of vertebrates. Many are viviparous. Important species include:

(*a*) *Wohlfartia vigil* (**the New World flesh-fly**). This species occurs in North America and often deposits its larvae in skin lesions, the eye or the nares, especially of children, causing disfiguring lesions and much suffering. *W. meigeni* has a similar distribution and habits.

(*b*) *W. magnifica* (**the Old World flesh-fly**). This species, also known sometimes as the sheep maggot-fly occurs in Southern Europe, the Mediterranean region and the Middle East. The larvae, which are deposited in open wounds and the nares, ears, eyes and vagina, cause serious lesions and disfigurement. It is an important cause of sheep myiasis in South Russia.

(*c*) *Sarcophaga* spp. These forms, which are of almost worldwide distribution, have similar habits to the preceding genera, but can also deposit their larvae on food or other organic matter. If

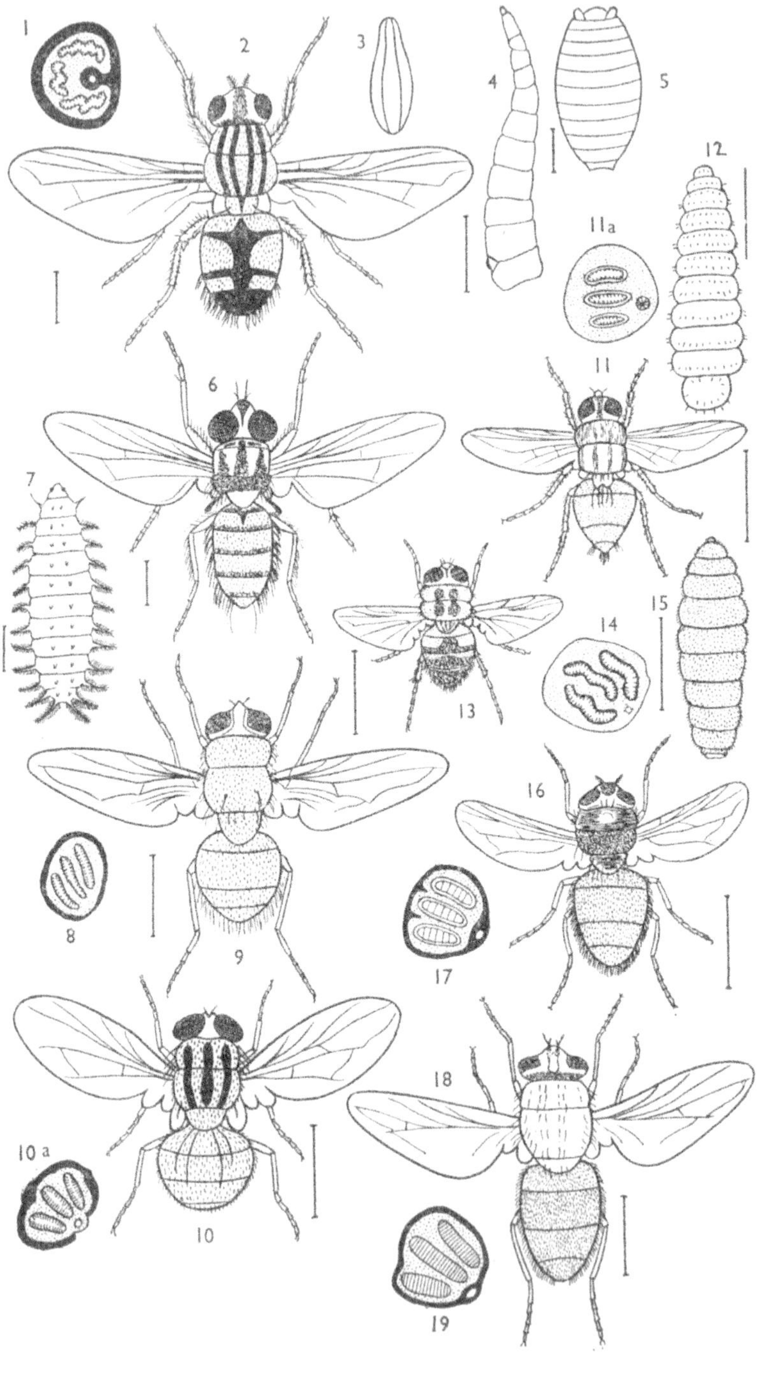

1
2
3
4
5
12
11a
6
11
7
15
14
13
16
8
9
17
18
10 a
10
19

such infested food is subsequently consumed by man or domestic animals the larvae are capable of becoming temporary parasites and of continuing their development in the bowel.

Oestridae (Bot- or Warble Flies)

These are large, hairy, variously coloured bee-like flies, the larvae of which are parasitic in warm-blooded vertebrates, chiefly mammals. The adults have reduced mouthparts and do not feed. Insect taxonomists distinguish several groups which are ranked as sub-families or even as families (Hypodermatidae, Gasterophilidae, Cuterebridae, etc.). Species of medical and veterinary importance include:

(*a*) *Dermatobia hominis* **(the tropical bot-fly).** This tropical American form captures a vector insect, usually a mosquito or filth-fly, and glues its eggs to the abdomen. When the vector alights on a suitable host the eggs become detached and adhere to the skin or hair. The peculiar, club-shaped larvae (**Macaw worms**), stimulated by the body warmth, emerge and burrow into the subcutaneous tissue, where they produce large, painful or itching, boil-like lesions. They eventually reach a length of 20–25 mm and then leave the host and drop onto the ground to pupate. The adult fly is bright blue. Man, cattle, pigs, dogs, cats, sheep, rabbits and various birds are suitable hosts, but not horses or mules.

(*b*) *Gasterophilus* spp. **(the horse bot-flies).** These forms attach their eggs direct to the hairs of the host, whence the hatched larvae are licked off and, adhering to the tongue, are transferred to the mouth. They make their way down to the stomach by tunnelling

FIG. 24. Non-bloodsucking Flies—I

1 *Musca domestica*—posterior spiracle of larva.
2 —adult fly.
3 —egg.
4 —larva.
5 —puparium.
6 *Fannia scalaris*—adult fly.
7 —larva.
8 *Chrysomyia bezziana*—posterior spiracle of larva.
9 —adult fly.
10 *Callitroga macellaria*—adult fly.
10a —posterior spiracle of larva.
11 *Auchmeromyia luteola*—adult fly.
11a —posterior spiracle of larva.
12 —larva.
13 *Cordylobia anthropophaga*—adult fly.
14 —posterior spiracle of larva.
15 —larva.
16 *Calliphora vomitoria*—adult fly.
17 —posterior spiracle of larva.
18 *Lucilia sericata*—adult fly.
19 —posterior spiracle of larva.

in the mucosa and submucosa of the tongue and buccal cavity, pharynx, oesophagus and stomach. Some occasionally go astray and reach other organs. In the stomach they emerge into the lumen and attach themselves to the wall, where they complete their larval development. When ready to pupate they drop off and pass down through the intestine and out through the anus onto the ground. Man becomes infected by handling horses and then shows the symptoms of gastric irritation; or he may acquire a skin infestation with the larvae tunnelling in the subcutaneous tissue.

(*c*) *Hypoderma* spp. (**the cattle bot-flies**). The eggs of this species also are attached by the females direct to the hairs of the host; but, on hatching, the larvae crawl down the hair to the skin, which they penetrate, and then undertake an extensive migration through the tissues of the host, eventually returning to the subcutaneous tissue in the region of the back. Here they produce inflamed swellings known as 'warbles' from which, after some time, they escape through a perforation and drop to the ground to pupate. Heavily infected cattle show poor growth and reduced milk yield, the migrating larvae causing great irritation to the surrounding tissue; and the hide is much damaged and often rendered commercially worthless by the formation of the warbles. In the relatively rare cases of human infection the larvae confine their activities to tunnelling in the subcutaneous tissues, causing a form of creeping eruption.

(*d*) *Oestrus ovis* (**the sheep bot-fly**). The viviparous females of this species deposit their larvae in the nares or eyes or on the lips of the host, whence they crawl into the nasal sinuses. When larval development is complete they emerge again and drop onto the ground to pupate. The larvae cause much irritation to the sheep so that they become restless and cease to feed. Emaciation and death are not uncommon in severe infections. In man the larvae burrow into the mucous membranes and the tissues surrounding the sinuses, causing painful and disfiguring ocular and nasal lesions. *O. ovis* is cosmopolitan in distribution.

(*e*) *Rhinoestrus purpureus* (**the Russian gad-fly**). This species closely resembles *O. ovis* in life-cycle and habits, but infects chiefly horses and cattle and occurs in Northern and Eastern Europe and Asia Minor. Human cases also occur from time to time. Pathogenesis in both animal and human hosts also resembles that due to *O. ovis*.

Oscinidae (Chloropidae) (The Eye-gnats)

These small (2–6 mm), smooth, black flies have short wings devoid of closed cells, and short antennae. The labella is spiny and forms a cutting instrument. The larvae normally feed on plants or in decaying vegetable matter and include several important plant pests. However, the genera *Hippelates* and *Siphunculina* are attracted by lachrymal and sebaceous secretions, blood and pus; and the larvae are therefore found in wounds and sores, and on mucous membranes, especially the conjunctiva. They cause some local irritation and spread conjunctivitis and trachoma.

Myiasis

Parasitism by dipterous larvae is characterised by local pain and pruritis. The lesions vary in gravity according to the size and number of parasites and according to whether they actually penetrate the tissues or only attach themselves to the surface. Nasal, aural and ocular forms—whether in man or animals—may be accompanied by extensive erosion of tissue with accompanying disfigurement and pain. Forms of subcutaneous myiasis in which the fly larvae excavate long tunnels are known as **creeping eruption** or **larva migrans.** They closely resemble the similar lesions produced by certain species of nematodes. Human intestinal myiasis, although not uncommon, is probably always accidental. It has been reported due to over twenty species including *Fannia canicularis*, *Musca domestica* and species of *Sarcophaga* and *Chrysomyia.*

Treatment usually involves surgical removal of the larvae, in man at least.

Control

Control of filth-flies involves:

(*a*) Prevention of breeding by sanitary disposal of human and animal faeces, stable refuse, garbage and decaying organic matter of all kinds.

(*b*) Destruction of larvae by treatment of breeding sites with insecticidal sprays.

(*c*) Measures directed against the adults, such as residual spraying of human and animal accommodation with insecticides, fumigation, and the use of traps and screens.

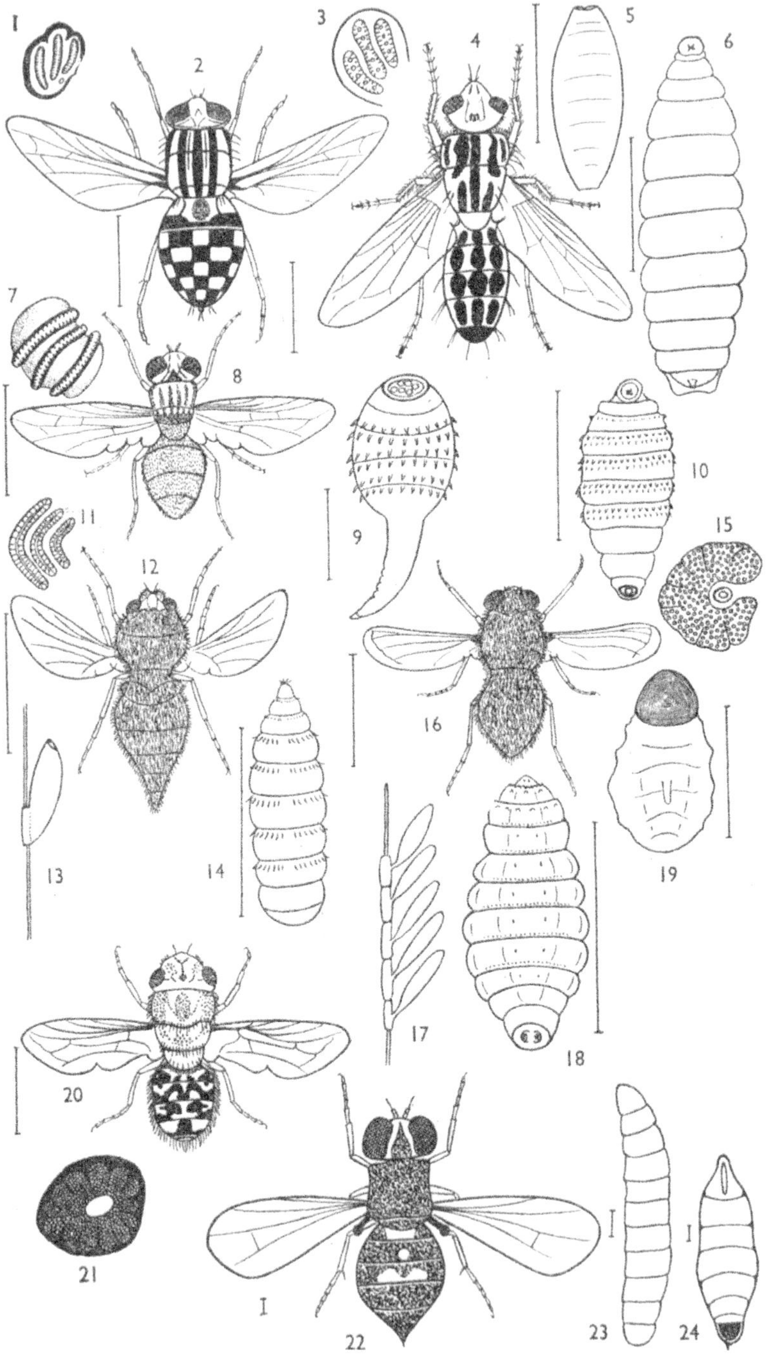
1
2
3
4
5
6
7
8
9
10
11
12
13
14
15
16
17
18
19
20
21
22
23
24

(*d*) Protection of human food and eating and drinking utensils by screening and covering.

Control of myiasis-producing flies involves:

(*a*) Cleanliness and regular disinfection of sleeping places of domestic animals.
(*b*) Treatment of animals with insecticides (dips, dusts or sprays) to kill the parasites on them or to render them less attractive to the parasites.
(*c*) Control of adult flies as above, where this is practicable.
(*d*) Treatment of all lesions and complete destruction of maggots found therein.
(*e*) Special methods, such as the feeding of systemic insecticides to stock, and the release of large numbers of male flies sterilised by irradiation to prevent breeding. The latter method has been claimed to produce dramatic success in eradicating the American screw-worm fly from Florida.

Among the great variety of insecticidal substances used may be mentioned DDT, gammexane, dieldrin, aldrin, malathion, diazinon, methyoxychlor, lindane, chlordane, ruelene, dimethoate and sodium arsenite; as well as a number of proprietary compounds. The organophosphorus compounds have been particularly successful in certain infections; and some of these can be administered to stock systemically.

FIG. 25. Non-bloodsucking Flies—II

1 *Sarcophaga haemorrhoidalis*—posterior spiracle of larva.
2 —adult fly.
3 *Wohlfahrtia vigil*—posterior spiracle of larva.
4 —adult fly.
5 —puparium.
6 —larva.
7 *Dermatobia hominis*—posterior spiracle of larva.
8 —adult fly.
9 —young larva (ver macaque)
10 —older larva (torcel)
11 *Gasterophilus intestinalis*—posterior spiracle of larva.
12 —adult fly.
13 —egg attached to hair of host.
14 —larva.
15 *Hypoderma bovis*—posterior spiracle of larva.
16 —adult fly.
17 —eggs attached to hair of host.
18 —larva.
19 —empty puparium after escape of fly.
20 *Oestrus ovis*—adult fly.
21 —posterior spiracle of larva.
22 *Hippelates pusio*—adult fly.
23 —larva.
24 —puparium.

LICE
(ANOPLURA AND MALLOPHAGA)

Two distinct orders of insects are included under this popular name, viz., the **Anoplura** or **Sucking Lice** and the **Mallophaga** or **Biting Lice.** Both are of medical and veterinary importance.

Anoplura

The members of this order are very small insects (1–2 mm). They are generally dark-coloured, wingless, tough-skinned, dorsoventrally flattened insects with short but conspicuous antennae and reduced eyes. The legs are modified for attachment to hairs by the reduction of the tarsus and the provision of special claws. The retractile mouthparts are of the piercing-sucking type. Sucking lice are obligatory ectoparasites of mammals, transferred from one host individual to another by contact and unable to live apart from the host for more than a few days. The eggs are attached by the female to the body hairs of the host and hatch rapidly, giving rise to young forms (nymphs) which closely resemble the adult except in size and lack of sexual maturity. The course of development involves three moults and occupies about two to three weeks. There is no metamorphosis. All stages feed on the blood of the host and discharge pellets of dark-red excreta. The species which attack man and domestic animals are as follows:

(*a*) *Pediculus humanus* (**head and body lice**). This species has two localised but freely inter-breeding forms, viz., *P. h. corporis* (**the body louse**) and *P. h. capitis* (**the head louse**).

(*b*) *Phthirius pubis* (**the crab louse**). This species infests the genital and inguinal regions and is transmitted during coitus.

(*c*) *Haemotopinus* spp. This genus includes *H. asini* of equines, *H. suis* of pigs and *H. eurysternus* and *H. quadripertusus* of cattle. The former is known as **the short-nosed cattle louse.**

(*d*) *Linognathus* spp. This genus includes **the blue lice of sheep** (*L. ovillus* and *L. africanus*) **the foot louse of sheep** (*L. pedalis*) and **the long-nosed cattle louse** (*L. vituli*), together with several other species parasitic on goats, dogs and foxes.

Human sucking lice are unpleasant ectoparasites which cause intense pruritis and transmit various spirochaetal and rickettsial infections, including relapsing fever, trench fever and typhus fever. Infestation is associated with poverty, filth and overcrowding, especially in cold climates. Personal hygiene is essential in preventing infestation. Delousing of infested clothing can be achieved by exposure to dry or moist heat, or by treatment with pediculicides (soaking in antiseptic solutions, fumigation with sulphur dioxide or methyl bromide, spraying with lethane 384 or benzyl benzoate, dusting with or soaking in solutions or suspensions of DDT or gammexane, etc.). Heat treatment is best because it also kills spirochaetes and rickettsiae. Mass delousing of infested persons is practised in army camps and special plant is available for this purpose. Individual treatment involves application of lotions or ointments containing pediculicidal substances (phenyl cellosolve, benzyl benzoate, DDT, benzocaine, etc.), followed by shampooing and fine combing. In severe infestations of head and crab lice it is necessary to cut the hair short or shave it off altogether. Sucking lice of domestic animals cause irritation and restlessness with resulting loss of condition; and some transmit other pathogens, such as swine fever. Milk production may fall in infested cattle.

Mallophaga

The members of this order are also very small insects. They differ from the Anoplura primarily in having biting mouthparts and in feeding on fragments of hair, feathers, skin scales and dried blood from scabs. It is now known, however, that in some of them the mouthparts are suctorial also and that they suck blood. None affect man but a number of species are troublesome ectoparasites of domestic animals, especially poultry:

(*a*) *Lipeurus heterographus*. This species is **the head louse of poultry** and is a dangerous parasite of fowl and partridge chicks.

(*b*) *Lipeurus caponis*. This species is **the wing louse of poultry.**

(*c*) *Goniocotes gallinae*. This very small form is known as **the fluff louse of poultry** and occurs in the fluff at the base of the feathers of pigeons, fowls and pheasants.

(*d*) *Goniodes* spp. *G. meleagridis* is **the common turkey louse** and *G. gigas* is **the giant body louse of poultry.**

(*e*) *Columbicola columbae*. This species is **the pigeon louse.**

(*f*) *Anaticola* spp. Several species of this genus parasitise ducks.

(*g*) *Trichodectes* spp. This large genus of mammal parasites has been divided by systematists into several smaller genera, but the important forms are still commonly known by their old names. Among them may be mentioned *T. bovis* of cattle, *T. equi* of horses, *T. ovis* of sheep, *T. caprae* and *T. limbatus* of goats and *T. canis* of

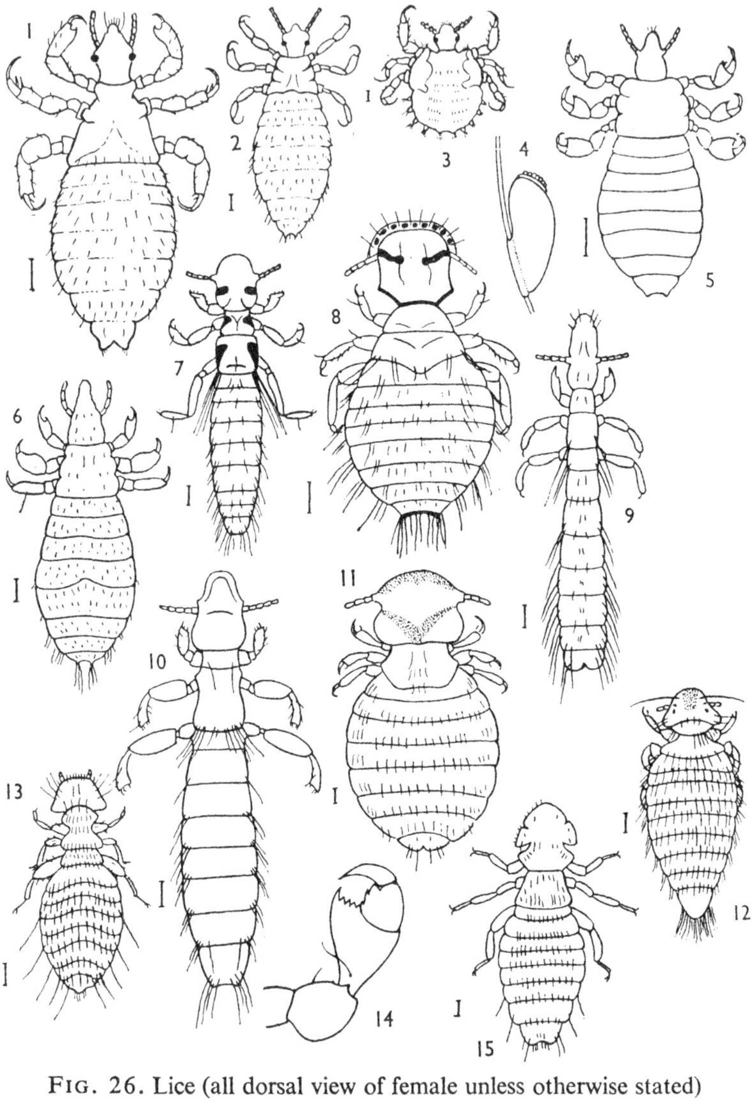

FIG. 26. Lice (all dorsal view of female unless otherwise stated)

1 *Pediculus humanus corporis*. (Human body louse.)
2 *Pediculus humanus capitis*. (Human head louse.)
3 *Phthirius pubis*. (Crab louse.)
4 Egg of *P. h. capitis* attached to human hair.
5 *Haematopinus eurysternus*. (Short-nosed cattle louse.)
6 *Linognathus vituli*. (Long-nosed cattle louse.)
7 *Lipeurus caponis*. (Wing louse of poultry.)
8 *Goniocotes gigas*. (Giant body louse of poultry.)
9 *Columbicola columbae*. (Pigeon louse.)
10 *Anaticola crassicornis*. (Duck louse.)
11 *Trichodectes canis*. (Biting louse of dogs.)

dogs. A closely related form—*Felicola subrostrata*—occurs on cats. *T. canis* is a vector of the dog tapeworm *Dipylidium caninum*.

(*h*) *Menopon gallinae*. **The shaft louse of poultry** parasitises fowls, ducks and pigeons, while a closely-related species occurs on peacocks. The eggs are laid on the feathers.

(*i*) *Menacanthus stramineus*. **The yellow body louse of poultry** occurs on the less densely feathered skin of the body of fowl, turkey, peacock and pheasant and is dangerous to young chicks.

(*j*) *Heterodoxus* spp. *H. spiniger* parasitises dogs in hot climates and other species of this genus occur on kangaroos and wallabies.

Biting lice, like sucking lice, cause irritation to their hosts, especially in cold weather, with resulting restlessness, biting and scratching, damage to hair or feathers and, in poultry, reduced egg production. A variety of insecticidal dusts, washes and dips have been used for control, including DDT, gammexane, lindane, rotenone, sodium fluoride and organophosphorus compounds. Nicotine fumigation in poultry houses is an effective method.

FLEAS

(SIPHONAPTERA)

These small, tough-skinned, laterally compressed insects belonging to the order Siphonaptera (Aphaniptera) are entirely wingless and have long hind-legs adapted for jumping. The eyes are reduced or lacking, the antennae short and sunk in grooves at the sides of the head, and the mouthparts of the piercing-sucking type. The body is provided with many backwardly directed hairs and short stout spines, the latter being often so regularly arranged as to resemble combs. They are active ectoparasites of warm-blooded animals and, like the lice, are specific in the choice of a host, although not to the same extent.

Metamorphosis is complete. The eggs are deposited in small batches in the nest, kennel or dwelling of the host, and hatch in a few days, giving rise to slender, cylindrical, whitish larvae with distinct head, antennae and biting mouthparts, but no eyes or legs.

---

12 *Menopon gallinae*. (Shaft louse of poultry.)
13 *Menacanthus stramineus* (Yellow body louse of poultry.)
14 Distal part of leg of *Haematopinus asini* (Sucking louse of equines) showing claw and tibial pad for grasping hair of host.
15 *Heterodoxus longitarsus*. (Tropical dog louse.)

They feed on the organic debris that they find about the sleeping quarters of the host and, when mature, spin a silken coccoon covered with an effective camouflage layer consisting of particles of dirt, inside which they pupate, eventually emerging as adults to attack fresh host individuals. The adult may remain as a resting stage inside the pupa case for long periods if no host is immediately available. Longevity depends on humidity and nutrition. Unfed fleas do not live long in dry surroundings. Well-fed fleas in humid conditions may live as long as three years.

A number of species are important parasites of man and his domestic animals, among which may be mentioned:

Pulex irritans (**the human flea**);
Xexopsylla cheopis, *X. astia* and *X. braziliensis* (**the tropical rat-fleas**);
Nosopsyllus fasciatus (**the temperate zone rat-flea**);
Ctenocephalides canis (**the dog-flea**);
C. felis (**the cat-flea**);
Synosternus pallidus (on rats, hedgehogs and mammals preying on them);
Leptosyllus segnis (**the cosmopolitan mouse-flea**, which also occurs on rats);
Ceratophyllus gallinae (**the chicken-flea**);
Echidnophaga gallinacea (**the sticktight-flea of poultry**, which also attacks dogs, cats, horses, rabbits, pigeons and ducks); and
Tunga penetrans (**the sand-flea, chigoe-flea or chigger**).

Pulex irritans, which is occasionally found also on rats and pigs, has decreased greatly in Europe in the last fifty years, but has spread to many parts of the tropics. Members of the genus *Xenopsylla* require a higher temperature in order to complete their development, and therefore exist in temperate climates only in heated buildings.

Fleas are important to man in two ways:

(1) **As Troublesome Ectoparasites**

Their bite may cause severe irritation in some persons and animals, which may be the result of an anaphylactic response following previous sensitisation. *Tunga penetrans*, the sand-flea, is particularly troublesome to man. Both sexes of this species at first live free in dry sandy soil, in the dust and ashes of dirty dwellings, and in the rubbish on the floors of ill-kept stables, byres and

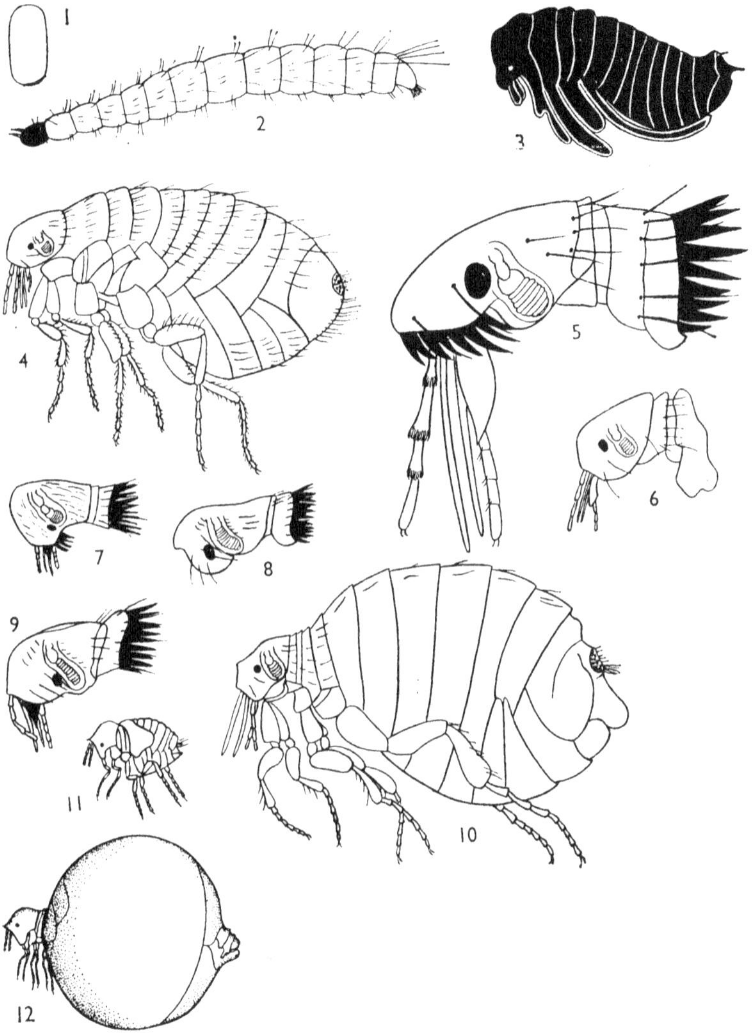

FIG. 27. Fleas

1 *Xenopsylla cheopis*—egg.
2 —larva (side view).
3 —pupa (side view).
4 —adult female (side view).
5 *Ctenocephalides felis*—head enlarged, to show eye, antenna, genal and pronotal combs, and mouthparts.
6 *Pulex irritans*—head (N.B.—no combs).
7 *Leptopsylla segnis*—head (N.B.—genal and pronotal combs).
8 *Ceratophyllus gallinae*—head (N.B.—pronotal comb only).
9 *Nosopsyllus fasciatus*—head (N.B.—pronotal comb only).
10 *Echidnophaga gallinacea*—adult female (side view).
11 *Tunga penetrans*—female before fertilisation.
12 —female after fertilisation and host-penetration, showing swollen abdomen filled with eggs.

poultry pens, and feed intermittently on the blood of any available warm-blooded animal. After fertilisation, however, the female attaches herself to the skin of the first warm-blooded animal encountered, usually attacking the feet, and burrows in deeply. In man the favourite sites are between the toes and at the roots of the nails. The body of the female, filled with eggs, swells up to the size of a pea, causing pain and irritation and often leading to serious secondary infection. When the eggs have been discharged the female dies and disintegrates. Originally a tropical American form (30° N to 30° S), *T. penetrans* spread to Africa about a century ago and has more recently become introduced into India. The sticktight-flea, *Echidnophaga gallinacea*, burrows in the skin of its avian hosts and oviposits there, producing swellings which ulcerate. The larvae fall out and develop on the ground. Both young and adult birds can be killed by heavy infestations.

(2) **As Vectors of Pathogens**

Fleas are primarily responsible for the spread of the following human infections, but are not known to be vectors of any important animal diseases:

Bubonic plague. This disease, caused by *Pasteurella pestis*, is spread by the rat-fleas *Xenopsylla cheopis*, *Nosopsyllus fasciatus* and *Synosternus pallidus* (and more rarely by *X. astia* and *X. braziliensis*), which often attack man. After taking blood from an infected host the flea may transfer bacilli to an uninfected host either:

(*a*) By regurgitating blood and bacilli into the puncture wound of another host individual, following interrupted feeding.

(*b*) By depositing faeces containing bacilli (which have multiplied in its intestine) near the puncture wound of a new host-individual, into which they will be inoculated by scratching.

(*c*) By wandering from host to host attempting to feed and being unable to do so because multiplication of the bacilli in the intestine of the flea has led to blocking of the proventriculus, but injecting some bacilli into the host at each attempt.

The last method is the most usual one.

Endemic murine typhus (Brill's disease). This malady is also spread by the rat-fleas *X. cheopis* and *N. fasciatus*, together with *X. astia*.

Hymenolepiasis diminuta. Infection with the rat tapeworm,

Hymenolepis diminuta, which readily establishes itself in man, is transmitted by *Ctenocephalides canis*, *Pulex irritans*, *Ctenopsyllus segnis*, *X. cheopis* and *N. fasciatus*, all of which are potential intermediate hosts of this parasite.

Dipylidiasis caninum. Infection with the dog tapeworm, *Dipylidium caninum*, which also readily establishes itself in human beings, especially children, is transmitted by *C. canis*, *C. felis* and *P. irritans*, the normal intermediate hosts.

Control

The control of fleas involves the following measures.

(1) Destruction of the adult insects by treatment of the hosts with insecticidal dusts, lotions or sprays; and cleanliness in the home and in all poultry houses, kennels, stables, byres and the like. DDT, gammexane, chlordane, lindane, diazinon, malathion, dimethoate and rotenone have all been found effective in the removal of fleas from their hosts and the destruction of larvae in their habitats.

(2) Insufflation of rat burrows with DDT powder or fumigation with gammexane smoke to kill the fleas before anti-rat measures are undertaken is always necessary, otherwise the fleas will leave the dead rats and attack human beings.

(3) Anti-rat measures, including fumigation of ships, rat-guards on mooring ropes, poisoning, trapping, and rat-proofing of buildings (especially food-stores) and garbage containers.

(4) Insecticidal treatment of houses that have been occupied by persons infected with bubonic plague.

(5) Cleanliness and insecticidal treatment of houses, stables, byres, pig and poultry pens and kennels in areas where sand-fleas are endemic, together with daily application of lysol-vaseline or other suitable repellent to the feet.

BUGS

(HEMIPTERA)

These insects belonging to the order Hemiptera vary in size from minute to very large. They have an incomplete metamorphosis, the immature forms or nymphs closely resembling the adults. The anterior pair of wings are stiff and thickened proximally but are thin and membranous distally; while the hind wings are uniformly thin and membranous, and are generally shorter and wider than the front pair. When folded and at rest, both pairs of wings lie horizontally over the back. In a number of species the wings are lacking. The long antennae have only four or five joints. Conspicuous compound eyes and usually also two or three simple eyes or ocelli are present on the head. The piercing-sucking mouthparts form a beak projecting forwards from the front end of the head. The majority feed on plant juices or small invertebrates; and the order consequently includes many species of agricultural importance. Two families only include members worthy of mention in connection with medical and veterinary science.

Reduviidae (Triatomidae) (Assassin Bugs)

These are large (1–4 cm by 0·25–1 cm), dorsoventrally flattened, oval, brown or black insects with a rigid, curved beak, functional wings and elongate legs. The nymphs are flightless but the adults of both sexes are powerful fliers. Most species are carnivorous and feed on other insects, but a few are ectoparasites and suck the blood of man and other mammals. The blood-sucking forms frequent human habitations, especially native huts, and infest the burrows of rodents and armadillos, feeding by night and hiding during the day in cracks and crevices. The medically important forms belong to the genera *Reduvius*, *Panstrongylus*, *Rhodnius* and *Triatoma*. All occur in the New World only, mainly in Central and South America, within the range 41° N to 41° S, with the exception of *T. rubrofasciata*, which is cosmopolitan. Many species inflict vicious bites, especially the common and notorious **kissing bug**, *Reduvius personatus*, (which possesses a salivary toxin and attacks the face, particularly the lips, whence its name), *Rhodnius prolixus* and *T. sanguisuga*, **the Mexican bedbug.** *P. megistus* and *T. infestans* are domestic species which transmit Chagas' disease (caused by *Trypanosoma cruzi*) and *T. rubrofasciata* is suspected of transmitting kala-azar (caused by *Leishmania donovani*) in India. When gorged with blood they defaecate near the wound, into which the infected faeces may subsequently be inoculated by scratching. Control is difficult, owing to the fact that reduviid bugs are resistant to DDT. Screening of houses and beds, cleanliness and the use of gammexane or dieldrin, have some effect. Dogs, foxes and cats are also often attacked.

Cimicidae (Bed-bugs)

In the members of this family wings are vestigial and ocelli lacking. The small (5 mm), tough-skinned, dark brown body is conspicuously flattened dorsoventrally, the head is short and sunk into the notched thorax up to level of the eyes, and the abdomen is almost circular in outline. The whole body is covered with thick-set short hairs. The large, bottle-shaped eggs are laid in batches in crevices and crannies in the woodwork of houses, in furniture especially beds and mattresses, and behind pictures. The nymphs resemble the adults but are lighter in colour. They mature in about six weeks, passing through four moults, if blood meals are available. Adults and immature forms alike are nocturnal in habits, hiding in crevices by day and coming out at night to attack their victims; feed only on blood; and are able to withstand starvation for extended periods. Nests can be located by finding the black faecal pellets around the holes. The species of medical importance are:

Cimex lectularius **(the European bed-bug).** This species of evil reputation has spread through most of the temperate areas of the world and has even invaded some tropical countries.

C. hemiptera **(the tropical bed-bug).** This form, also known as *C. rotundatus*, occurs in the warmer parts of the world, especially in rural areas.

Leptocimex boueti **(the West African bed-bug).** This restricted species is of considerable local importance.

Bed-bugs are principally noxious on account of their bites, which are harmless to some people but produce severe pruritis with local oedema and inflammation in others, leading to insomnia and neurasthenia. Experimentally they are capable of transmitting a wide range of pathogenic organisms but do not appear to act as vectors under natural conditions. Control can be effected by the use of moist heat, to which they are very sensitive; fumigation with hydrocyanic acid gas, trichloracetonitrite, or sulphur dioxide; treatment of cracks in walls and furniture with oil-soap emulsion; and the use of sprays or dusts containing DDT, gammexane, malathion or diazinon. The organophosphorus compounds are highly toxic to human beings, however, and beds and sleeping quarters, especially of young children, should not be treated with them. Some members of this family are important parasites of poultry, notably *Haematosiphon inodora*, **the Mexican chicken-bug,** *Ornithocoris toledoi*, **the Brazilian chicken-bug,** and several species of *Cimex*. These forms attack fowls, turkeys and pigeons, causing severe irritation and anaemia.

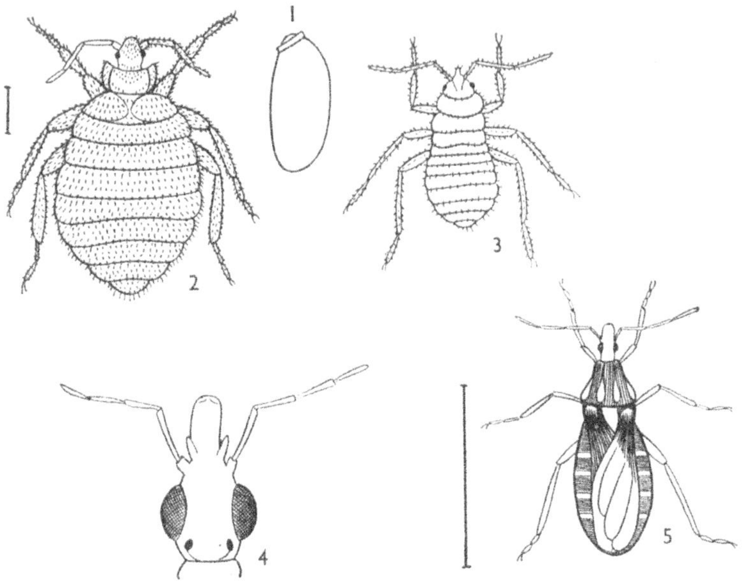

FIG. 28. Bugs (Hemiptera)

1 *Cimex lectularius* (bed-bug)—egg.
2 —adult.
3 —nymph.
4 *Panstrongylus megistus*—head.
5 —entire adult.

OTHER INSECT GROUPS

Larvae and adults of certain species of beetles (Coleoptera), moths (Lepidoptera) and grasshoppers and cockroaches (Orthoptera) act as intermediate hosts for some of the helminth parasites of man and domestic animals.

Bees, wasps and hornets, and certain species of ants can inflict a venomous sting on man and his animals, which can be dangerous or even lethal if the attackers are numerous. Some species of ants can inflict a venomous bite.

MITES AND TICKS

(ACARINA)

These small to microscopic arachnids have a compact, ovoid, unsegmented body in which the head, thorax and abdomen are fused and indistinguishable; four pairs of usually six-jointed legs;

mouthparts consisting of a pair of pedipalps, a pair of chelicerae and a median structure known as the hypostome; and a membranous or leathery integument which may be strengthened by chitinous plates or shields dorsally and ventrally. Simple eyes are present in some species. The mouthparts are attached to a movable anterior part of the body known as the capitulum, the whole being referred to as the gnathosoma. The gnathosoma is often attached to the rest of the body by a hinge. The majority have a tracheal respiratory system. In most species there hatches from the eggs a six-legged larval form known as a hexapod larva. This stage feeds and moults into an eight-legged nymph which also feeds and eventually moults into the sexually mature adult. There may be more than one nymphal stage. The following orders contain representatives of medical and veterinary importance;

Demodicoidea (Follicular Mites)

The members of this sub-order have a very small, elongate, annulate body; three-jointed legs; and a single pair of spiracles opening usually near the base of the capitulum. Eyes are lacking. They occur in the hair follicles or sebaceous glands of mammals. *Demodex folliculorum* infests man. It rarely causes discomfort unless unusually numerous, when it may produce dry, chronic erythrema with burning irritation and scaling of the epidermis. The mites are transmitted mechanically or by direct contact. Youth, debility and skin diseases are predisposing factors. Other species of this genus infest cats and dogs, sheep and goats, cattle and pigs. In animals secondary infection with pyogenic bacteria may take place and the resulting lesions are much more serious than the original infestation, sometimes leading to emaciation and death.

Parasitoidea (Parasitoid Mites)

These are very small leathery mites, often provided with shields or plates; lacking eyes; and having stylate chelicerae. The spiracles are carried on lateral chitinous plates above or behind the base of the third pair of legs. The majority are parasitic on various vertebrate and invertebrate hosts, but some species are free-living and carnivorous. Several species normally parasitic on other hosts attack man if opportunity offers.

Dermanyssus gallinae **(the chicken mite).** This form sucks the blood of poultry at night, hiding in crevices during the day. If numerous they cause irritation and anaemia resulting, in avian hosts, in listlessness and reduced egg-production. It has been alleged that this species can transmit encephalitis of man and horses; but this remains unconfirmed.

Ornithonyssus sylviarum (**the northern poultry mite**). The habits and pathogenic effects of this species are similar to those of *D. gallinae.* It attacks poultry in temperate climates, and occasionally man and other mammals. Unconfirmed reports suggest that it can transmit fowl pox and human and equine encephalitis.

O. bursa (**the tropical fowl mite**). Common on fowls and pigeons in the warmer parts of the world, this species will also attack man. It remains on the host, causing similar effects to the two preceding species.

Liponyssus bacoti (**the tropical rat mite**). The female lays her eggs in the nests and burrows of the rats and the nymphs and adults drop off the host after each blood meal. *O. bacoti* is the intermediate host of the filarial parasite of rats, *Litomosoides carinii,* which is widely used in experimental work on filariasis.

Allodermanyssus sanguineus (**the house mouse mite**). This parasite of the common house mouse is believed to transmit *Rickettsia akari,* the cause of rickettsialpox in man.

Pneumonyssus caninum (**the nose mite of dogs**). This mite inhabits the nasal passages and sinuses of dogs but does not penetrate any further down the respiratory tree. It causes nasal irritation resulting in sneezing and head-shaking.

Sarcoptoidea (Itch Mites, Mange Mites, Hair-clasping Mites and Feather Mites)

These are very small, soft-bodied mites, lacking both eyes and tracheae. Suckers and hooks may be present on the legs and suckers may also occur at the genital opening or near the anus. The legs are supported beneath the integument by rods (epimera). Several families are parasitic on mammals and birds, including man and his domestic animals;

SARCOPTIDAE (Sarcoptic Itch and Mange Mites)

These are short-legged, globose mites which burrow deep in the skin of their hosts, the females laying their eggs in the tunnels thus excavated. On animal hosts they usually attack those areas of the body which are not hirsute. The result of their activities is the production of intense irritation; and the resulting scratching and rubbing causes inflammation, thickening of the skin and scab-formation. The following species are important:

Sarcoptes scabiei. This species produces **scabies** in man; and related species of the same genus cause **sarcoptic mange** in dogs and cats, sheep and goats, cattle and horses, pigs and fur-bearing mammals.

Cnemidocoptes gallinae. This species produces **depluming itch** in fowls by burrowing into the skin beside the shafts of the feathers, causing irritation and inflammation so that the feathers break off.

C. mutans. This species attacks the feet and legs of fowls and turkeys, causing the condition known as **scaly leg.**

Notoedres cati. This species attacks cats and rabbits, especially the skin in the region of the ears and the back of the neck.

PSOROPTIDAE **(Psoroptic Itch and Mange Mites)**

These are longer-legged, oval mites which remain at the surface of the skin of their hosts and prefer those areas of the body which are well-covered with wool or hair. The eggs are laid on the skin at the edges of the lesions. Progessive scab lesions are formed as a result of the mites' activities, the wool or hair falls out in the affected areas, and the constant irritation leads to interference with feeding followed by emaciation and death. Man is not normally attacked by psoroptic mites. The following species are important:

Psoroptes spp. (**psoroptic mange mites** *sensu stricto*). The validity of the numerous described species of this genus is suspect at the present time. Suffice it to say that species or strains or races attack sheep, goats, cattle, horses and other equines, and rabbits. The form which causes **sheep-scab,** an important disease now virtually eradicated from Britain, is often known as *P. ovis.*

Chorioptes spp. (**chorioptic mange mites**). Like the preceding genus, the alleged species of *Chorioptes* are now suspect by acarologists. Although capable of infesting any area of the skin, they are most frequently found on the legs and in the ears. Horses, sheep, goats, cattle and rabbits are the principal host species. The form which causes **itchy leg** or **foot mange** in horses in often known as *Ch. bovis.*

Otodectes cynotis (**the otodectic mange mite**). This species attacks the ears of dogs, cats and fur-bearing mammals. In severe infestations, if the disease is not checked, purulent inflammation of the external ear develops, which may extend to the middle and inner ear and brain, with very serious effects.

CYTODITIDAE (CYTOLEICHIDAE) **(Tissue Mites of Birds)**

One species is of veterinary importance, namely, *Cytodites nudus*, sometimes known as **the air-sac mite,** which lives in the respiratory passages and air-sacs of fowls, turkeys and pheasants. It is not, apparently, very pathogenic unless infestation is very heavy.

LISTROPHORIDAE **(Hair-Clasping Mites)**

These mites have laterally compressed bodies and their legs and pedipalps are modified for clasping the hairs of their hosts. They occur on small mammals, notably the rabbit, the guinea-pig and the smaller fur-bearers.

ANALGESIDAE, DERMOGLYPHIDAE and PROCTOPHYLLIDAE **(Feather Mites)**

These three families live on or in the feathers of various avian hosts, including fowls, pheasants, peacocks, pigeons and turkeys. In general they are not particularly pathogenic, but may occasionally cause a mild form of depluming itch if infestation is severe.

Tarsonemoidea (Predaceous Mites, Plant Mites and Grain Mites)

These are very small, soft-bodied mites having the body distinctly divided into cephalothorax and abdomen; needle-like chelicerae; and the legs arranged in two groups, two pairs being placed far forward and two pairs far back. The spiracles open on the ventral surface of the body. *Pediculoides ventricosus*, **the North American grain itch mite,** normally feeds upon the larvae of insects infesting grain and straw; but it will attack man if opportunity offers, burrowing in the skin and causing an annoying form of dermatitis.

Trombidoidea (Harvest Mites, Red Mites, Velvet Mites, Chiggers)

The members of this sub-order have a hairy body clearly divided into cephalothorax and abdomen; spiracles opening at the sides of the capitulum; and the terminal joint of the pedipalps chelate and adapted for grasping. The larvae are blood-suckers, the adults and nymphs are free-living in soil. The larvae of many species attack man, causing severe **dermatitis,** although the normal hosts are rodents, birds, snakes, turtles and toads. The eggs are laid on the ground and the emerging larva attaches itself to the first suitable host available. The irritation caused by the bites of the larva results in scratching and rubbing which, in turn, may be followed by secondary infection and the formation of necrotic ulcers. Certain species, particularly members of the genus *Trombicula*, are also of importance in veterinary medicine.

Trombicula autumnalis (**red spiders**). The larvae of this species attack not only man but also all types of domestic animals. They are commoner on chalky soils than on clay and are initially deep red in colour. The itching which they cause in man can be almost intolerable. It has been suggested that they may be the cause of **heel-bug** of race-horses.

T. akamushi and *T. deliensis*. These species, which occur in Southern Asia and the Far East, are the vectors of scrub typhus (Tsutsugamushi disease or Japanese river fever) caused by *Rickettsia orientalis* (*R. tsutsugamushi*).

T. sarcina (**blacksoil itch mite**). This mite, which occurs in the true black earth areas of Australia, normally parasitises kangaroos and wallabies. However, it readily attacks man, dogs, sheep and horses. In Queensland it is the cause of the disease of sheep known as **blacksoil itch** or **leg itch.**

T. minor (**Queensland scrub-itch mite**). This species attacks man, although the normal hosts are rodents.

T. alfreddugesi (**common red bug**). This species ranges throughout the Americas, being apparently commonest in the U.S.A. It will attack almost any vertebrate host; and, in man, produces the most severe lesions where the body is constricted by clothing.

Neo-schöngastia americana. This mite attacks poultry in North and Central America and a related species occurs in Japan and the Pacific Islands. Affected birds fetch lower prices.

Tyroglyphoidea (Cheese and Grain Mites)

These very small, pale, fat, soft-bodied mites usually lack eyes. The cephalothorax and abdomen are usually distinct, the chelicerae prominent and the pedipalps small. Tracheae and therefore spiracles are lacking. Some species have a hard-skinned, short-legged, migratory stage, known as a **hypopus**, which lacks a mouth and is provided with ventral suckers for attachment to the insects and small mammals by which it is disseminated. The hypopus moults into an octopod nymph. The majority feed on such organic products as cheese, flour, cereals, hay and feathers, or on decaying vegetable matter; but a few species may penetrate the superficial layers of the human skin, especially in persons handling infested

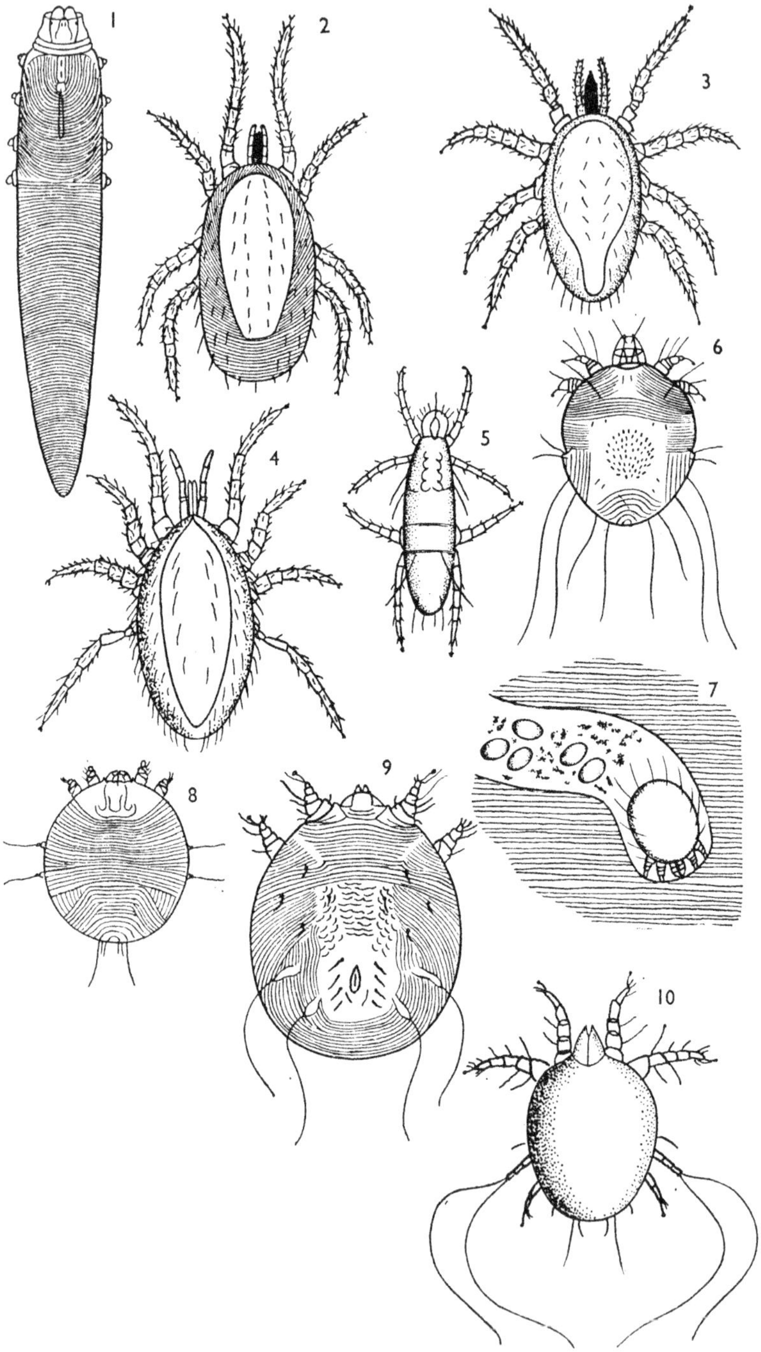
1
2
3
4
5
6
7
8
9
10

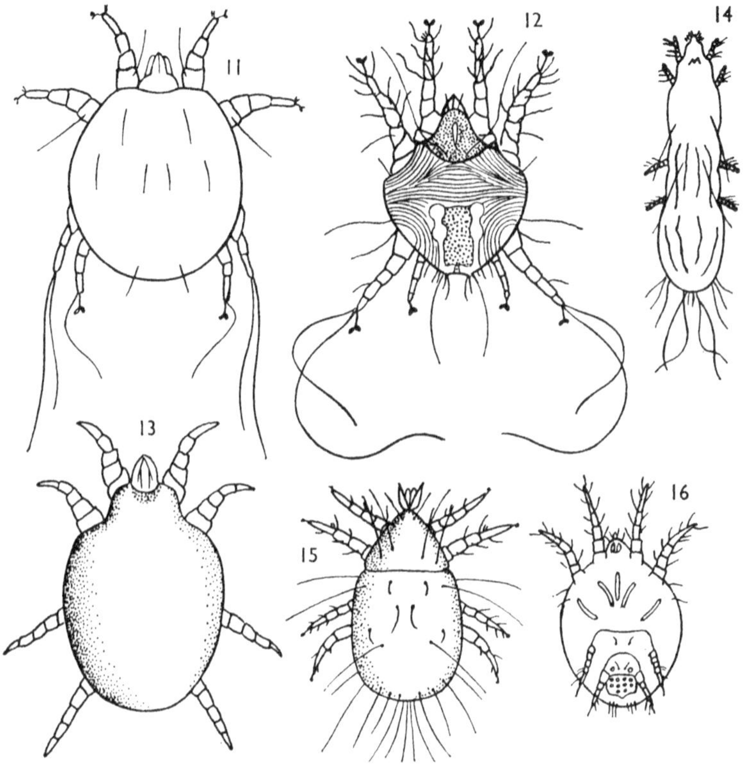

FIG. 29. Mites (all dorsal view unless otherwise stated)

1 *Demodex folliculorum*—adult male (females are about two-thirds length)
2 *Dermanyssus gallinae*—adult female.
3 *Ornithonyssus sylviarum*—adult female.
4 *Liponyssus bacoti*—adult female.
5 *Pediculoides ventricosus*—adult female.
6 *Sarcoptes scabei*—adult female.
7 —adult female burrowing in skin and leaving elliptical eggs and faecal debris in her wake.
8 *Cnemidocoptes gallinae*—adult female.
9 *Notoedres cati*—adult female.
10 *Psoroptes ovis*—adult female.
11 *Chorioptes bovis*—adult female.
12 *Otodectes cynotis*—adult male.
13 *Cytodites nudus*—adult female.
14 *Syringophilus columbae*—adult female.
15 *Tyroglyphus longior*—adult female.
16 Travelling larva (hypopus) of *Tyroglyphus*—ventral view showing suckers.

products, and cause an itching **dermatitis** variously known as **grocer's itch, coolie itch, copra itch,** etc. Cheese mites may be swallowed and appear in the faeces, causing transient diarrhoea if numerous.

Oribatoidea (Beetle Mites)

Although containing no parasitic members, this sub-order is of importance inasmuch as the tapeworms of the family Anoplocephalidae all utilise various species as intermediate hosts. These mites are small free-living forms found amongst vegetation and vegetable debris, on which they feed. They have a hard exoskeleton (hence the popular name) and are provided with specialised setae at each posterior corner of the cephalothorax.

Ixodoidea (Ticks)

The members of this sub-order, all of which are blood-sucking ectoparasites, are large, ovoid acarines, differing from the mites of the other sub-orders in having an armed hypostome, leathery integument and conspicuous capitulum. The spiracles open on chitinous plates behind the coxae of the third and fourth pairs of legs. The young larval stages live on the ground or amongst vegetation and await the passing of a suitable host, to which they attach themselves to feed. When full-fed the larva moults to become a nymph; and the nymph, in turn, after engorging with blood, moults to become an adult or imago. Finally, the adult female, after engorging, drops off the host and lays her eggs on the ground. Newly-hatched larvae are known as seed-ticks. Male ticks die after mating. With respect to the life-cycle, ticks fall into three groups, namely, (*a*) those which require three hosts, because they drop off after engorgement and moult on the ground; (*b*) those which require two hosts, because the larva moults on the host while the nymph drops off to moult on the ground; and (*c*) those which require but a single host, since all three stages engorge on the same individual. These are known respectively as three-host, two-host and one-host ticks. Various modifications of this basic life-cycle occur. Some species have two or more nymphal stages, for example, and in some the adults do not feed. There are two important families.

Argasidae (Soft Ticks)

These forms have no hard dorsal shield; the capitulum is ventral to the anterior extremity; the spiracles are behind the third pair of legs; and blood is taken twice or more in each stage of the life-cycle, the female ovipositing after each feed except in those species in which the adults do not feed at all, when oviposition may continue intermittently for months. There is often more than one nymphal stage. Adult males and females scarcely differ in their external features. The following are important parasites of man and domestic animals:

Argas persicus **(the fowl tick).** This species is a common parasite of all kinds of domestic and many wild birds; and also attacks man. The irritation resulting from the bites makes the birds restless at night, egg production drops sharply, and anaemia may develop due to loss of blood. This tick may also cause a form of paralysis in ducks and transmits piroplasms and spirochaetal infections of fowls.

Otobius megnini **(the spinose ear tick).** This species attacks principally the ears of dogs, sheep, cattle and horses; but goats, pigs, cats, rabbits and man are not immune. Irritation due to the bites of these ticks results in inflammation and secondary infection, which may be serious. The external auditory meatus may be packed with the parasites.

Ornithodoros moubata **(the eyeless tampan).** This tick, although able and willing to feed on almost any vertebrate host available, seems to have become adapted to man and his domestic animals in Africa, where it frequents native huts and the vicinity of human dwellings. It transmits fowl spirochaetosis; has been cited as a vector of Q fever; and is the only natural vector of African relapsing fever, caused by the spirochaete, *Borrelia duttoni.*

O. savignyi **(the eyed tampan).** This species attacks camels, fowls and other domestic animals in India, the Middle East and Africa. It occasionally bites man.

Ixodidae (Hard Ticks)

These forms have a hard dorsal shield or scutum, which covers the whole back of the male but only the anterior part of the back in the larva, nymph and female; the capitulum extends forward from the anterior extremity; the spiracles are behind the fourth pair of legs; and blood is taken only once in each stage of the life-cycle, the female laying but a single batch of eggs. The following members of this family are important in human and veterinary medicine.

Ixodes spp. Almost every kind of domestic animal is attacked by one or more species of this genus; and man himself is not immune. The following deserve mention:

I. ricinus **(the common European dog tick or castor-bean tick)** Although most frequent on dogs, this species also occurs on other domestic animals. It transmits pyaemia of young lambs in Britain, an infection caused by *Staphylococcus aureus*; encephalitis; Q fever; haemorrhagic fever; the virus infection louping ill and the rickettsial tick fever of sheep; red-water fever of cattle and sheep due to *Babesia bovis*, this piroplasm being passed through the eggs from one generation of ticks to the next; and canine piroplasmosis.

I. hexagonus **(the hedgehog tick).** This British form also attacks dogs and fur-bearing mammals.

I. canisuga **(the British dog tick).** This species attacks not only dogs, but also horses and sheep. It may be very troublesome in kennels and is a potential menace on silver fox farms.

I. pilosus **(the russet tick or bush tick).** This species occurs on sheep and goats, cattle, horses, pigs, cats and dogs in South Africa.

I. rubicundus **(the South African paralysis tick).** This is another South African form which occurs on cattle, sheep and goats, causing tick paralysis. It is susceptible to dry heat and therefore found in moist areas, chiefly in winter.

I. holocyclus **(the Australian paralysis tick).** This species occurs on human beings, dogs and cats, and other domestic animals in the coastal bush and scrub areas of Australia and Tasmania, causing tick paralysis.

Haemaphysalis spp. This genus of rather small ticks has several important species:

H. leachi **(the dog tick).** This form is widely distributed in the southern hemisphere, occurring on cats, dogs and fur-bearing mammals in Africa, Asia and Australia. It transmits canine piroplasmosis, tick bite fever and Q fever.

H. leporis-palustris **(the rabbit tick).** This is a very common form in North and South America, where it attacks not only rabbits but also various birds, cats, small fur-bearers and wild rodents, and also man. It transmits Q fever, Rocky Mountain spotted fever and tularemia, the infection passing through the eggs of the tick from one generation to another.

H. cinnabarina. This species occurs in North and South America where it attacks poultry. The subspecies *H. c. punctata* is Asian and European in distribution and attacks sheep and goats, cattle and horses, and rabbits, as well as a wide variety of wild hosts. It causes tick paralysis in cattle and sheep and transmits various piroplasms.

Amblyomma spp. The numerous species of this genus are large and broad. The following are important:

A. americanum **(the lone star tick).** This species, which infests cattle in the southern and eastern U.S.A., in Mexico and in northern South America, owes its name to the single silvery spot which ornaments the scutum of the female. It transmits Rocky Mountain spotted fever and possibly also Q fever.

A. maculatum **(the Gulf Coast tick).** This North American species is a serious pest of cattle, which it predisposes to attack by the screw-worm fly, *Cochliomyia hominovorax*.

A. cajennense. This species attacks man, cattle, horses and dogs in the southern U.S.A., Central America and South America. It transmits São Paulo fever.

A. hebraeum **(the bont tick).** This South and Central African form attacks all domestic animals, especially cattle, sheep and goats; and occasionally infests man. It is a serious pest of cattle in South Africa. It transmits heart-water fever of sheep, goats and cattle and human African tick typhus.

A. variegatum **(the variegated tick).** This is another African parasite of cattle and sheep, which transmits Nairobi sheep disease, heart-water fever and Q fever.

Dermacentor spp. This genus of usually rather ornate ticks also includes some species of major importance:

D. andersoni **(the wood tick).** This North American form attacks cattle, sheep and horses principally; but also dogs, cats and pigs; rabbits and wild rodents; and sometimes man. It causes a serious form of tick paralysis and transmits Rocky Mountain spotted fever and tularemia to man, encephalomyelitis to horses, various piroplasms and Q fever. Infection passes through the eggs of the tick.

D. variabilis **(the American dog tick).** This is also a North American species. It attacks principally dogs, but occurs also on all other domestic animals, many wild forms, and man. It transmits Rocky Mountain spotted fever, encephalitis, tularemia and various piroplasms, as well as being a cause of tick paralysis.

D. reticulatus. This South European and Asian form attacks all domestic animals.

Hyalomma aegyptium **(the bont leg tick).** This species occurs widely in Africa, Asia and Southern Europe, where it attacks chiefly cattle, but also sheep, goats, cattle, dogs, cats, rodents and birds, including poultry. It may occasionally attack man. *Theileria* spp., the cause of East Coast fever in cattle and several species of *Rickettsia* are transmitted by this form, including the causative organisms of African tick typhus, tick-bite fever and possibly Q fever. Other species of the genus *Hyalomma* also act as vectors of these and other infections.

Rhipicephalus spp. This genus contains a large number of species, many of which are important vectors of infectious diseases. Among them may be mentioned the following:

R. sanguineus **(the brown dog tick).** This species is found in almost all the warmer regions of the globe, and attacks chiefly dogs, being often established in kennels. However, it also occurs on horses, camels, cats and the larger fur-bearers; and occasionally attacks man. It is a proven vector of canine piroplasmosis (biliary fever), *Babesia* infections of dogs and horses, *Rickettsia* infections of domestic animals and man, including Q fever and tick-bite fever; and of a number of viral diseases, including Nairobi sheep disease. It is not only one of the most important and dangerous acarine vector species, but also causes tick paralysis in dogs.

R. appendiculatus **(the brown ear tick).** This African species occurs mainly south of the equator, where it attacks cattle, sheep and goats, equines and, more rarely, dogs, attaching itself to the areas under the tail and in the ears. It transmits East Coast fever of cattle caused by *Theileria parva*, of which it is the chief vector, tick-bite fever, exanthematic fever of dogs, *Babesia* infections of cattle, Nairobi sheep disease and louping ill. In the case of *Babesia bigemina* the infection passes through the egg of the tick.

R. evertsi **(the red-legged tick).** This species occurs in Africa south of the equator on many domestic animals and has been incriminated in the transmission of spirochaetoses of cattle, sheep and goats, and horses; red-water fever of cattle; East Coast fever of cattle; tick-bite fever; and biliary fever of horses. The infective agent in the first two diseases mentioned, namely, *Borrelia theileri* and *Theileria parva*, are passed via the eggs from one generation of ticks to another.

Boophilus annulatus **(the North American cattle tick).** This species attacks cattle, sheep and goats in North America, where it transmits red-water fever, the causative organism—*Babesia bigemina*—passing from one generation of ticks to the next through the eggs.

Several other species of this genus, including the notorious **blue tick** (*B. decoloratus*) of Ethiopia, attack cattle, sheep, goats, horses, pigs and dogs in various parts of the world and transmit red-water fever and gall-sickness of cattle, Q fever and various spirochaetoses.

Margaropus winthemi (**the Argentine tick).** This South American tick occurs on horses principally and is one of the few members of this family which have not so far been incriminated in the transmission of some disease of man or his animals. It has recently been introduced into South Africa.

It is clear from the above account of their activities that ticks are pathogenic in three ways. Firstly, their bite is painful and irritating, causing local inflammatory reaction. Secondly, they are capable of producing a condition known as **tick paralysis** in sheep, cattle, dogs and man, due to the injection of neurotropic salivary toxins, particularly if their bite is in the neighbourhood of the spinal column. Death may follow owing to paralysis of the respiratory muscles. Thirdly, they act as vectors of a wide range of human and animal infections, among them the viral diseases Colorado tick fever, several forms of encephalitis, Nairobi sheep disease, tick-bite fever and louping ill of sheep; the rickettsial diseases Rocky Mountain spotted fever, Mediterranean boutonneuse fever, the forms of typhus known as African tick fever and Russian tick fever, heart-water disease of sheep, goats and cattle, and Q fever; the bacterial and spirochaetal diseases relapsing fever and tularaemia, anthrax, brucellosis, and various spirochaetoses of cattle, sheep, goats, equines and poultry; and the protozoal diseases red-water fever of cattle (Texas cattle fever), European cattle fever, piroplasmoses of dogs, equines and sheep, haemorrhagic fever of sheep, goats and horses, and anaplasmosis of sheep and cattle.

Prevention and control of ectoparasitosis due to acarines varies according to the types involved. So far as man is concerned, the wearing of protective clothing impregnated with DDT, benzyl benzoate, dimethyl or dibutyl phthallate, or the use of repellents containing such substances, clearing of grass and bush (since the mites are very sensitive to drying and sunlight), and the spraying of infested areas with gammexane or other acaracides, are among the measures recommended against trombiculid mites. Personal and group hygiene and avoidance of over-crowding are important against sarcoptid mites. Avoidance of infested areas and materials

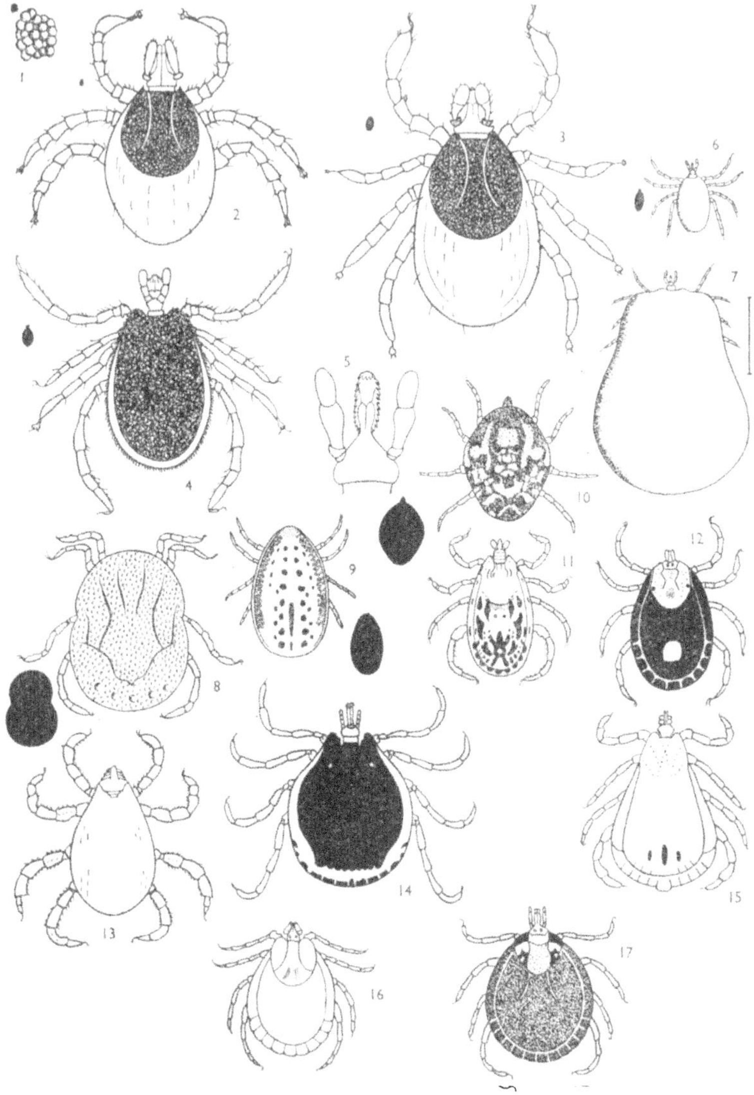

FIG. 30. Ticks

1 *Ixodes ricinus*—eggs.
2 —larva.
3 —nymph.
4 —adult male.
5 —capitulum with pedipalps and hypostome.
6 —normal female before engorgement.
7 —normal female after engorgement.
8 *Ornithodoros moubata*—adult female.
9 *Argas persicus*—adult female.
10 *Otobium megnini*—adult female.

is essential in the case of other mite infestations. Treatment involves the application of ointments or lotions containing such acaricidal substances as sulphur, pyrethrum, rotenone and gammexane. The control of soft ticks involves fumigation or burning of infested human habitations, stables, byres and poultry houses. Where this is not possible repeated pressure spraying with gammexane is often effective. The control of hard ticks involves destruction of wild hosts, especially rodents; destruction of vegetation that affords shelter for the ticks, their young stages or their rodent reservoir hosts—by razing or burning on wild land, by sheep grazing or extension of arable areas on cultivated land; disinfestation of domestic animals by the use of ixodicidal dips such as DDT, gammexane and various organophosphorus compounds; the use of tick-proof clothing by human beings obliged to enter infested areas; and the encouragement of natural enemies such as birds, mice and parasitic hymenopterous insects.

PENTASTOMIDA

(TONGUE-WORMS)

These are unsegmented, worm-like arthropods, highly specialised for parasitic life. They have a whitish, elongate, flattened or cylindrical body, consisting of a short cephalothorax and a long, annulate, tapering abdomen. The mouth is armed with a pair of retractile chitinous hooks for penetration and anchorage. There is a rudimentary alimentary tract, but respiratory, circulatory and excretory organs are lacking. The sexes are separate. All stages are blood-sucking endoparasites of vertebrates, the adults living in the respiratory tract and the immature stages in the gut, viscera or body-cavity of their hosts. Some forms have a direct life-cycle and are innocuous so far as man is concerned. Other have an indirect life-cycle, larval infection being acquired by ingestion of raw vegetation contaminated with the nasal secretions of the definitive host, adult infection by consumption of the infected intermediate host. The majority live in reptiles, birds, fishes and small mammals;

---

11 *Dermacentor andersoni*—adult male.
12 —adult female.
13 *Boophilus annulatus*—adult male.
14 *Hyalomma aegyptium*—adult male.
15 *Rhipicephalus sanguineus*—adult male.
16 *Haemaphysalis concinna*—adult female.
17 *Amblyomma hebraeum*—adult female.

but a few species are of occasional veterinary and medical importance.

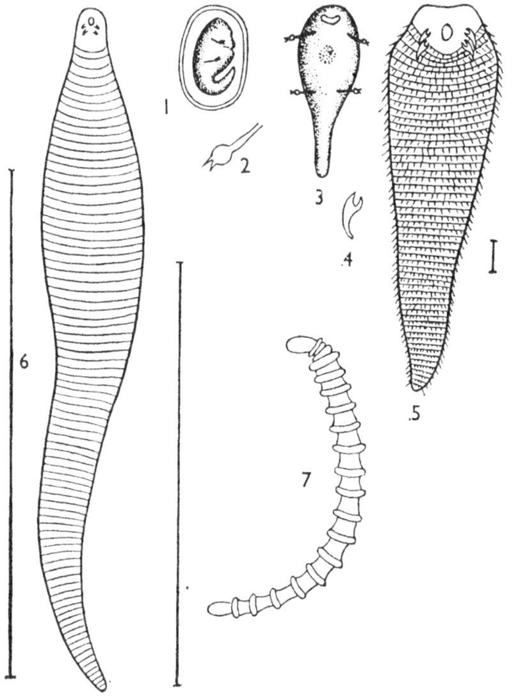

FIG. 31. Tongue-worms

1 *Linguatula serrata*—egg containing embryo.
2 —appendicular hook of newly-hatched larva.
3 —newly-hatched larva.
4 —fang (mouth-hook) of nymph.
5 —nymph.
6 —adult female.
7 *Porocephalus armillatus*—adult female.

Linguatula serrata is a relatively common cosmopolitan parasite the larvae of which are up to 5 mm in length and live in the viscera of rabbit, sheep, horse, goat and other herbivores; while the much larger adults (2–13 cm) infect the nasal cavities of dogs, wolves, foxes and, more rarely, horses and goats. Human infection with both adults and larvae occurs, the latter being more common.

Species of the genus *Porocephalus* occur as larvae in rodents and other herbivorous domestic and wild animals, as adults in various species of snakes. Human infection is sometimes reported and is probably more frequent than the records indicate, since the consumption of raw snakes forms an integral part of magical ceremonies indulged in by certain Central African tribes.

VENOMOUS ARTHROPODA

Members of four arthropod groups are capable of inflicting a venomous bite or sting of varying severity on man and domestic animals.

Insecta—Hymenoptera

Female bees, wasps and hornets and some kinds of ants inject venom through the modified ovipositor or sting, which is provided with special poison glands. Some other kinds of ant inflict a poisonous bite with their mandibles. The tropical fire-ant, *Solenopsis germinata*, is most dreaded on account of its burning, almost intolerably painful sting. Local pain and inflammation are usually the only symptoms, but systemic effects may follow in sensitised persons.

Myriapoda—Chilopoda

The large centipedes of warm climates can inflict painful and serious bites, causing local necrotic lesions accompanied by lymphangitis, fever, vomiting and headache. Death occasionally follows in children. The species of the genus *Scolopendra* are notoriously dangerous.

Arachnoidea—Scorpionida

All species of scorpions are potentially injurious to man, and some are very dangerous, the most serious effects being produced in young children, in whom a high fatality rate occurs. The sting, which is carried at the end of the abdomen, injects a toxalbumin. Both local effects (oedema and excruciating pain lasting for several hours) and systemic symptoms (muscular pains, headache, giddiness, nausea and vomiting, profuse perspiration, cold extremities and feeble pulse) are produced. In fatal cases death is due to respiratory paralysis.

Arachnoidea—Araneida

Most spiders are innocuous to man, but a few species can inflict a painful bite. The Tarantula of Southern Europe (*Lycosa tarantula*) and the Black Widow of North and South America (*Latrodectus mactans*) together with other species of the same genera, may be mentioned. The venom is again a toxalbumin and the effects are similar to those of scorpion sting, but less severe.

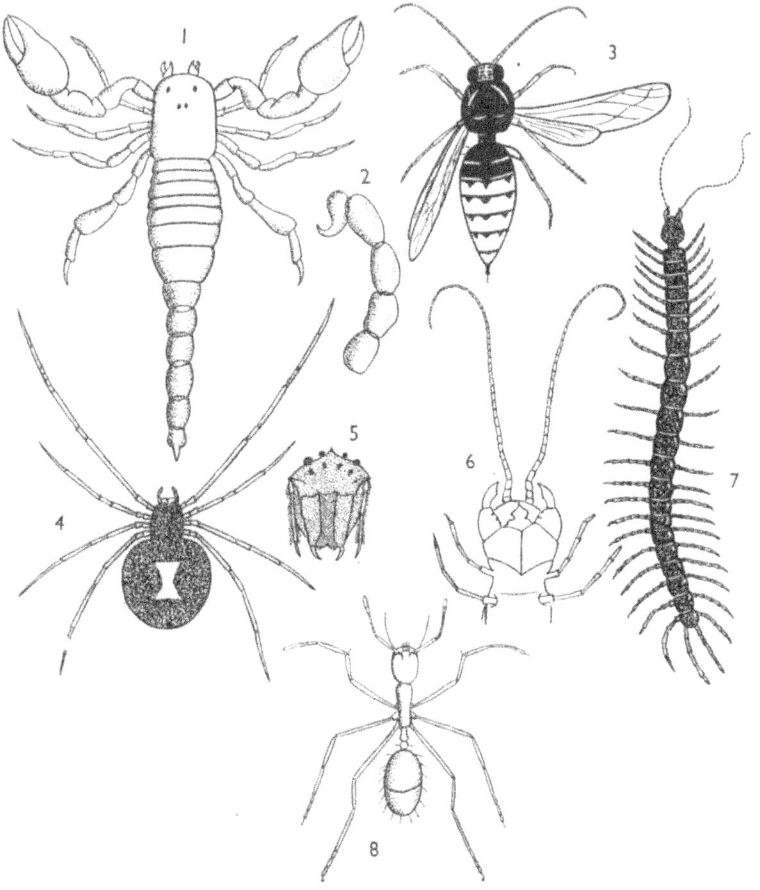

FIG. 32. Venomous Arthropods

1 Scorpion (dorsal view).
2 Terminal abdominal segments of scorpion in side-view to show telson and sting.
3 Hornet (*Vespa crabro*).
4 Black Widow Spider (*Latrodectus mactans*) (dorsal view).
5 Black Widow Spider (front view of head showing eyes and fangs—chelicerae).
6 Giant Centipede (*Scolopendra* sp.). Head, showing poison fangs and antennae.
7 Giant Centipede—from above.
8 Fire Ant (*Solenopsis*).

The majority of these venomous forms are carnivores which normally use their poison to kill or paralyse their prey. Lack of space forbids any further discussion of their characteristics. Domestic cleanliness is the most important control measure, but DDT and other insecticides can be used with good effect; and residual spraying is advisable in dwellings in warm climates. Treatment involves incision of the wound and irrigation with potassium permanganate; local application of ammonia or an anti-histaminic drug; injection of novocaine (or morphine in severe cases) to relieve pain; anti-shock treatment; and injection of antitoxic serum, if available.

CRUSTACEA

No member of this group is of direct importance as a cause of human or animal disease, but several act as biological or mechanical vectors. Thus small crustaceans of the widely distributed copepod genus *Cyclops* serve as intermediate hosts of the guinea worm, *Dracunculus medinensis*, the broad fish tapeworm, *Diphyllobothrium latum*, and species of the spiruroid nematode genus *Gnathostoma*. Species of the related copepod genus *Diaptomus* can also serve as intermediate hosts of *D. latum*. Larger crustaceans, such as the fresh-water crabs of the genera *Potamon*, *Eriocheir*, *Sesarma*, *Parathelphusa* and *Pseudothelphusa*, and the fresh-water crayfish of the genera *Astacus* and *Cambarus*, act as second intermediate hosts of the lung-fluke *Paragonimus westermani*. The crayfish *Potamobius* is a possible intermediate host of the acanthocephalan worm *Polymorphus boschadis*. The fresh-water shrimp *Gammarus pulex* and the water-louse *Asellus aquaticus* and the water-flea *Daphnia pulex* also serve as intermediate hosts of various spiruroid and acanthocephalan worms. In Kenya a phoretic association exists between fresh-water crabs of the species *Potamonautes niloticus* and the larvae and pupae of the blackflies *Simulium neavei* which transmit onchocerciasis.

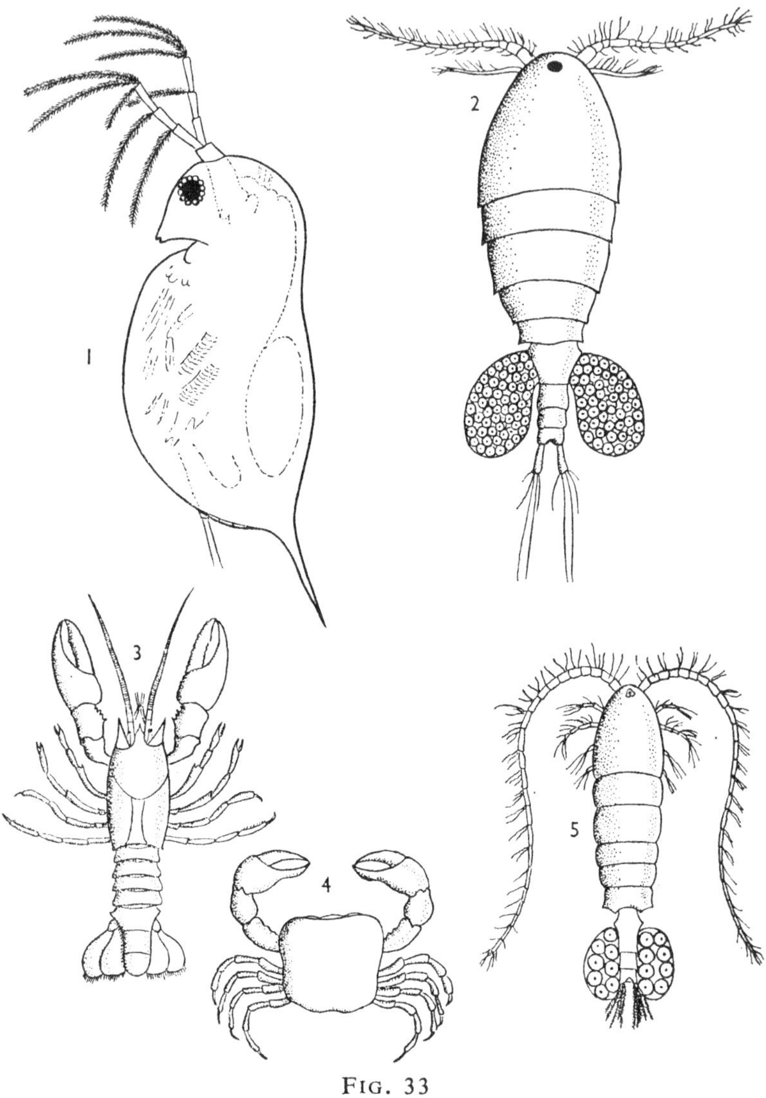

FIG. 33

1 *Daphnia* sp. (side view).
2 *Cyclops* sp. (dorsal view). Female with egg sacs.
3 *Cambarus* sp. (dorsal view).
4 *Potamon* sp. (dorsal view).
5 *Diaptomus* sp. (dorsal view). Female with egg sacs.

CHAPTER 5

MALACOLOGY

GENERAL

With the increasing realisation of the importance of the diseases of man and animals caused by parasitic trematodes, the study of the molluscan intermediate hosts which are invariably involved has now developed to the point where it has become an independent discipline. For medical and veterinary malacology, as for other branches of parasitology, special training courses now exist and openings are available for specialists.

The study of the anatomy, physiology, classification and ecology of even the relatively restricted group of molluscs which serve as biological vectors of the parasitic flukes is too vast a subject for any extended treatment in a work of this scope. However, so many references have been made to the molluscan intermediate hosts in the section on the trematodes that some further information is desirable.

CLASSIFICATION OF MOLLUSCS

The phylum Mollusca is subdivided into five principal classes, namely, the Amphineura or Chitons, the Scaphopoda or Tusk Shells, the Gastropoda or Slugs and Snails, the Pelecypoda (Lamellibranchia) or Bivalves and the Cephalopoda or Squids and Octopus. Of these, only the gastropods are important to the medical or veterinary parasitologist. The five classes are distinguished readily by the nature of the foot and of the shell. In the Amphineura the foot is flat and broad and the shell consists of eight dorsal plates or else both organs are altogether lacking; in the Scaphopoda the foot is conical and the shell tubular; in the Gastropoda the foot is again flat and broad, but the shell is a single spiral structure or may be lacking or embedded in the mantle; in the Pelecypoda the foot is shaped like a plough-share and the shell consists of two lateral valves hinged dorsally; while in the Cephalopoda the foot is drawn out into eight or ten long, powerful muscular tentacles, each bearing suckers, and the shell is lacking or reduced to a 'cuttle-bone' embedded in the mantle.

The Gastropoda include not only the slugs and snails but a number of other forms as well, the class being subdivided as follows:

Prosobranchia

In these forms the nervous system has been twisted by visceral torsion into a figure of eight; the mantle cavity opens anteriorly; there is usually a well-developed shell; and breathing is by gills (ctenidia). There are two orders in this sub-class, one of which contains important intermediate host species:

(*a*) Aspidobranchia (limpets, abalones, slipper shells, periwinkles and giant conch shells, etc.). The heart has two auricles and the ctenidia are plume-like with two rows of filaments. None are of medical or veterinary importance.

(*b*) Prosobranchia (cowries, whelks, cone shells, oyster drills and many kinds of fresh-water snails). The heart has only one auricle and the ctenidia have but a single row of filaments. The following families contain genera and species that are vectors of trematode infections:

Thiaridae (*Melaniidae*). *Semisulcospira* spp. and *Thiara* spp. are intermediate hosts of *Paragonimus westermani*; and the former also harbour *Metagonimus yokogawai*, while the latter also harbour *Clonorchis sinensis*. The snails *Cleopatra* and *Hua* also belong to this family. *Melania*, which often occurs in the literature, is a synonym of *Thiara*; and *Melanoides* and *Tarebia* are subspecies of this genus.

Pleuroceridae. *Goniobasis silicula*, the intermediate host of *Troglotrema salmincola*, belongs to this family.

Potamididae. This family of brackish water forms includes the intermediate hosts of *Heterophyes heterophyes*, namely, *Pirenella conica* in the west and *Cerithidea cingulata* in the east.

Pilidae (*Ampullaridae*). *Pila* spp., the second intermediate hosts of Garrison's fluke, *Echinostoma ilocanum*, belong to this family; as do also the genera *Turbinicola*, *Pomacea* and *Ampullarius*.

Synceridae (*Assimineidae*). A snail belonging to this family—*Syncera lutea*—is erroneously quoted in some texts as an intermediate host of the human lung fluke.

Viviparidae. *Viviparus javanicus* also serves as a second intermediate host of Garrison's fluke.

Bulimidae (*Bythynidae*, *Amnicolidae*). This family contains the notorious *Oncomelania* spp., the intermediate hosts of *Schistosoma japonicum*. In addition, *Alocinma longicornis* and *Parafossarulus manchouricus* are intermediate hosts of *Clonorchis sinensis*, as are also species of the genus *Bulimus* (= *Bythinia*). The last-named serve as intermediate hosts of the closely-related *Opisthorchis tenuicollis*. *Pomatiopsis lapidaria* is also said to harbour the human lung fluke, *P. westermani*. This family includes only fresh-water snails; but it is sometimes included with the very similar group of marine snails known as the Rissoidae.

Littorinidae. *Littorina pintado* harbours a cercaria capable of causing schistosome dermatitis.

Nassidae. *Nassa obsoleta* also serves as host to dermatitis-causing cercariae.

Opisthobranchia

In these forms the viscera and nervous system have become secondarily unwound; the mantle cavity opens posteriorly; the shell is usually absent, reduced or internal; and breathing is by gills or through the skin. None are of medical or veterinary importance. The sub-class includes such forms as the bubble shells, sea-slugs, sea-hares and the pelagic swimming molluscs known as pteropods.

Pulmonata

This sub-class includes the air-breathing fresh-water and land snails, and slugs. The mantle cavity opens anteriorly on the right and is provided with a vascular lining in order that it may serve as an air-breathing lung; gills are generally lacking; and, like the opisthobranchs but unlike the prosobranchs, these forms are all hermaphrodite. The following families contain genera and species that are of medical and veterinary importance:

Helicidae. *Cochlicella acuta* is a proven first intermediate host of *Dicrocoelium dendriticum*; and species of the genera *Euomphalia*, *Helicella* and *Theba* are also alleged to serve in this capacity.

Enidae (*Chondrinidae*). *Zebrina detrita*, *Ena obscura* and *Abida frumentum* are alleged to serve as first intermediate hosts of *D. dendriticum*.

Cionellidae (*Cochlicopidae*). *Cionella lubrica* (syn. *Cochlicopa lubrica*) is the proven first intermediate host of the lanceolate fluke, *Dicrocoelium dendriticum*.

Lymnaeidae. This large family contains many common species of great importance as intermediate hosts of trematode parasites. The genus *Lymnaea*, with its many subgenera (*Fossaria*, *Galba*, *Pseudosuccinea*, *Radix*, *Stagnicola* and *Myxas*), provides the intermediate hosts of the sheep liver fluke—*Fasciola hepatica*—and other closely related forms, and also many of the cercariae responsible for schistosome dermatitis.

Physidae. Species of the genus *Physa* also harbour schistosome dermatitis cercariae of various types.

Bulinidae. This family includes the genus *Bulinus*, with its subgenus *Physopsis*, members of which serve as intermediate hosts of the human blood fluke—*Schistosoma haematobium*—and related species of the same genus. By some authorities this family is included in the Planorbidae (q.v.).

Planorbidae. So far as human medicine is concerned, this family is the most important of all. It includes the genera *Hippeutis* and *Segmentina*, hosts of *Fasciolopsis buski*; *Biomphalaria*, *Australorbis* and *Tropicorbis*, hosts of *Schistosoma mansoni*; *Indoplanorbis exustus*, host of *Schistosoma spindale*; *Gyraulus* spp. and *Hippeutis umbilicalis*, both hosts of *Echinostoma ilocanum* and *Fasciolopsis buski*; and *Planorbarius metidjensis*, the host of *Schistosoma haematobium* in Europe.

Ancylidae. The fresh-water limpet, *Ferissia tenuis*, alleged host of *Schistosoma haematobium* in India, belongs to this family.

BIONOMICS AND CONTROL

In order to devise efficient methods for the reduction or elimination of populations of snail intermediate hosts in any given area, it is necessary to study the habits and ecological relationships of the species involved in great detail and over a considerable period of time. Climatic and seasonal factors, chemical and physical conditions in the habitat, food and feeding habits, breeding season, fecundity, life-cycle, and the effect of enemies and diseases are some of the matters which need to be investigated.

Much effective control can then generally be exercised by environmental methods, that is to say, by modification of the conditions which the snails find favourable. Since this is also generally beneficial to agricultural productivity in the area, the heavy costs involved can be more easily borne. Each snail species and each area forms a separate problem, however closely the situations in two different cases may appear to resemble each other. In particu-

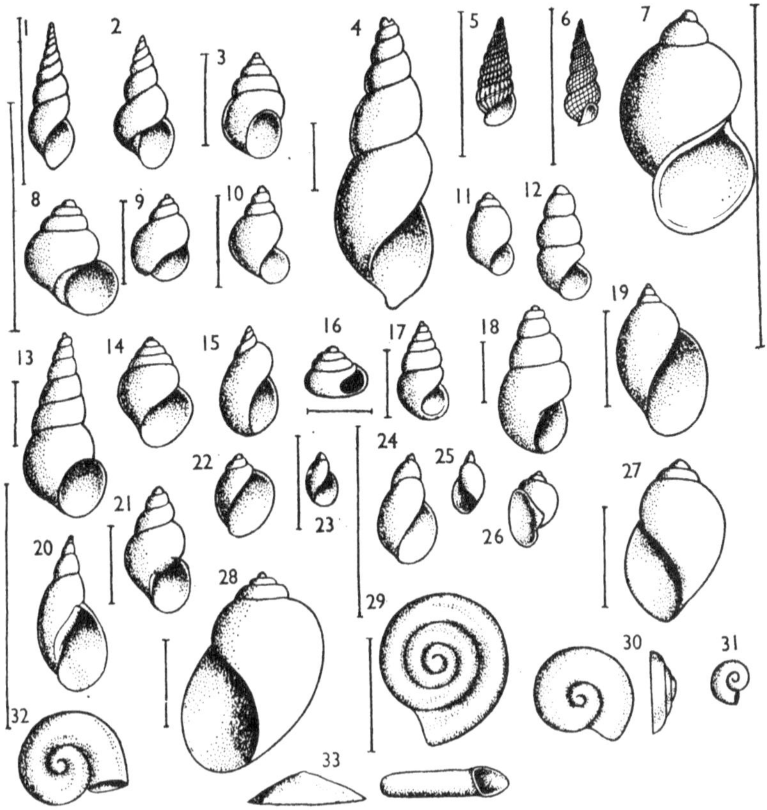

FIG. 34. Snails

1 *Thiara tuberculata.*
2 *Semisulcospira libertina.*
3 *Cleopatra* sp.
4 *Goniobasis silicula.*
5 *Cerithidea cingulata.*
6 *Pirenella conica.*
7 *Pila luzonica.*
8 *Viviparus javanicus.*
9 *Bythinia* (= *Bulimus*) *leachi.*
10 *Bythinia* (= *Bulimus*) *fuchsianus.*
11 *Alocinma longicornis.*
12 *Parafossarulus manchouricus.*
13 *Oncomelania nosophora.*
14 *Littorina pintado.*
15 *Nassa obsoleta.*
16 *Helicella itala.*
17 *Zebrina detrita.*
18 *Cionella lubrica.*
19 *Lymnaea natalensis.*
20 *Lymnaea stagnalis.*
21 *Lymnaea truncatula.*
22 *Myxas ampulla.*
23 *Radix ovata.*
24 *Stagnicola palustris.*
25 *Physa gyrina.*
26 *Physa parkeri.*
27 *Physopsis africanus.*
28 *Bulinus truncatus.*
29 *Biomphalaria alexandrina.*
30 *Segmentina hemisphaerula.*
31 *Gyraulus sp.*
32 *Indoplanorbis exustus.*

lar, very different methods of environmental control are required for amphibious snails, such as the members of the genus *Oncomelania*, and true aquatic snails, such as the bulinids and planorbids.

Where environmental control is not possible, resort has to be made to the application of molluscicides. Much progress has been made in this field in recent years. Originally copper sulphate was almost the only substance employed; but it has now been joined by less toxic and more effective compounds, such as the pentachlorophenates of sodium and copper, aqualin, 2-cyclohexyl-4,6-dinitrophenol (DNCHP), triphenyl tin acetate, iso-butyltriphenylmethylamine (ICI24223) and 5-chlorosalicylic acid-(2-chloro-4-nitro) anilide (Bayer 73 or Bayluscicide).

The work of the malacologist is to identify the species of mollusc serving as intermediate hosts of the parasite involved, to study its distribution and bionomics, and then to devise practicable and effective control measures directed against it. With the exception of the snail hosts of the sheep liver fluke, the major part of the work done in this field has been directed against the molluscan intermediate hosts of human trematode parasites.

CHAPTER 6

DIAGNOSIS, TREATMENT AND PREVENTION

DIAGNOSIS

Owing to the variability of the signs and symptoms, the frequency of multiple infection and the clinical resemblance between parasitic and non-parasitic diseases, diagnosis depends primarily upon laboratory findings. Any practical treatment of this subject would be out of place in the present volume, but mention may appropriately be made of some of the principal methods employed.

Examination of Faeces

Not only intestinal parasites but many which inhabit other parts of the body (lung-flukes, schistosomes) give rise to eggs or cysts which leave the host in the faeces. Direct microscopical examination of faecal smears in sometimes employed, but is tedious and unreliable except in very heavy infections. Methods for the concentration of cysts and ova include sedimentation, centrifugation, flotation using brine, centrifugal flotation using zinc sulphate solution and the acid-ether techniques which combine clarification of mucus, fatty material and faecal detritus with concentration. Quantitative methods include the filtration-count technique and Stoll's dilution-count technique.

Examination of Blood

Trypanosomes, malaria parasites, microfilariae and other blood-inhabiting forms are revealed by the microscope in thin or thick blood films, appropriately stained. Quantitative methods involve the used of ruled counting chambers. For microfilariae concentration of the blood by sedimentation or centrifugation is sometimes valuable. Romanovsky stains are most frequently employed.

Examination of Sputum

Direct microscopic examination of sputum smears can reveal eggs of lung-flukes and schistosomes, hydatid hooklets and membrane, and juveniles of *Ascaris lumbricoides*, *Strongyloides stercoralis*, hookworms, and other forms of which the migration route takes them through the lungs. Concentration by centrifugation may be carried out if the sputum has been previously diluted with 3 per cent sodium hydroxide solution.

Collection and Examination of Peri-anal Deposits

Human infection with thread-worms is most easily diagnosed by finding the characteristic ova with the microscope in material collected from the peri-anal skin. A wide variety of devices has been used for this purpose, among the best known of which are the National Institute of Health (N.I.H.) swab, the glass pestle, the brush and the adhesive cellophane swab. The last-named is consistently the most reliable.

Examination of Urine

Diagnosis of *Schistosoma haematobium* infection is generally made by finding the characteristic eggs in urine. Smears for inspection under the microscope are made following concentration by sedimentation or centrifugation.

Examination of Material from Lesions

In certain cases material from the actual lesions is most likely to reveal evidence of the parasite, particularly in skin infections such as oriental sore, creeping eruption and scabies.

Examination of Biopsy Material

Biopsied material obtained from the rectum, liver, spleen or other organs often reveals traces of adult parasites, their cysts or ova, when other methods have failed; as in kala-azar. Staining and microscopic examination are usually necessary.

Culture Methods

The presence of certain protozoan species (*Leishmania*, *Entamoeba*, *Trypanosoma*) can sometimes be confirmed by culture methods and a number of media have been devised for this purpose. Samples of soil, water, sewage, urine or faeces believed to contain ova of schistosomes, echinostomes, liver- or lung-flukes, or certain tapeworms, may be cultured in water or on moist filter paper so as to bring about hatching of the ova, when the active larvae are readily detected in a strong beam of light. Juvenile hookworms and *Strongyloides stercoralis* can be reared by mixing the soil or faeces containing the ova with an equal equantity of water and sterile sand or powdered charcoal in Petri dishes.

Xenodiagnosis

Confirmation of the presence of a particular parasite may sometimes be obtained by infecting susceptible experimental animals with material from the patient, as when reduviid bugs are fed on the blood of persons suspected of being infected with *Trypanosoma cruzi*.

Serological Methods

In general, serological methods are not so useful in parasitic infections as in bacterial and viral infections, owing chiefly to the difficulty of obtaining satisfactory antigens, the frequency of cross-reactions between different species, and the common occurrence of false positive and false negative results. They are therefore resorted to only when other techniques have failed to reveal positive evidence of the presence of the suspected parasite. Agglutination, precipitation, flocculation and complement fixation tests have been devised for amoebiasis, trypanosomiasis, leishmaniasis, malaria, toxoplasmosis, hydatid disease, schistosomiasis, trichinelliasis and the filariases. Circumlarval precipitate tests are occasionally employed in trichinelliasis, ascarid and strongyloid infections. Certain non-specific flocculative and chemical tests have been devised based upon the fact that disequilibrium of the serum proteins occurs in many parasitic diseases. Among these may be mentioned Henry's test and the protein-tyrosine test for malaria, Napier's formol-gel test and Chopra's antimony test for kala-azar and Sia's euglobulin precipitation test. Intradermal reactions are employed in the case of trichinelliasis, schistosomiasis and hydatid disease; and these, with the complement fixation test for the same infections, are the most often used and the most reliable of the serological reactions.

TREATMENT

The treatment of parasitic infections is, in general, based on the use of specific chemotherapy, a field in which great advances have been made during the last few decades. Since the early days of the war there has been a vast expansion in the volume of research directed to the discovery of new, less toxic and more effective and specific parasiticidal drugs. Extensive screening programmes have resulted in the discovery of many new weapons which can be effectively used against human and animal parasites. In a volume of this scope and purpose it would be out of place to go into detail, but among the more outstanding discoveries may be mentioned the broad-spectrum anthelmintic dithiazanine, the plasmodicides mepacrine and daraprim, the oxyuricide piperazine, the ascaricidal and hookworm-lethal bephenium salts, the schistosomicidal miracils, the amoebicidal iodohydroxyquinolines and the insecticides DDT, gammexane, and the organophosphorus compounds. Early parasiticidal drugs tended to suffer from the disadvantages of multiple dosage, frequent or severe toxic side-effects and slight disparity between dangerous and effective dosage level. The modern trend is towards drugs which are effective in a single dose (or in very few); which can be administered orally; which produce no side-effects; and which are not toxic, even in doses far exceeding those normally employed in therapy.

PREVENTION

The prevention of parasitic diseases and infestation depends primarily upon a knowledge of the life-cycle of the parasite and, in particular, of the mode of transmission and of the environmental factors which affect it. Preventive measures require to be aimed at interrupting the life-cycle of the parasite at some point. This may be achieved by treatment of the principal host to kill the adult stage; by environmental measures directed against free-living immature stages; by destruction of the intermediate hosts, if any; or by the prevention of transmission from host to host.

Therapeutic Prophylaxis

This involves the mass treatment of all infected persons or animals, so that the source of infection is eliminated.

Destruction of Reservoir Hosts

Although rarely possible, this is a logical extension of the principal of eliminating the source of infection.

Destruction of Intermediate Hosts

This is often the simplest and most effective way of preventing transmission. It is the principal measure employed in the prevention of schistosomiasis, fascioliasis and other snail-transmitted diseases; and in the prevention of parasitic infections transmitted by blood-sucking insects, such as malaria, trypanosomiasis and the filariases.

Destruction of Free-Living Stages

This measure is generally bound up with the following one, but specific steps of this kind are taken in certain cases as, for example, the destruction of larval trematodes by storage of infested water and the sterilisation of soil containing free-living helminth juveniles by application of superheated steam or chemicals, or by burying the topsoil.

Sanitary Disposal of Excreta

Since the eggs or cysts of almost all intestinal parasites and some non-intestinal forms leave the body of the definitive host in the faeces, the prevention of promiscuous defaecation and the sanitary disposal of faeces is a major step in the prevention of transmission. The use of human faeces (night-soil) as fertiliser, unless previously sterilised, also requires to be avoided. In the case of animal faeces these measures, though desirable, are rarely possible. In the prevention of human infection with urinary schistosomiasis, prevention of promiscuous urination into water is important.

Prevention of Dust Dispersal

Certain protozoan cysts and helminth ova are sufficiently resistant to desiccation to remain viable for considerable periods of time in dust, especially if the atmosphere is humid. Dust is therefore a source of infection and must be controlled, particularly in institutions.

Provision of Safe Drinking Water

Since infection with the Guinea worm is normally acquired by ingestion of the infected intermediate host in drinking water, and infective stages of many other parasites can be acquired in this way, the provision of potable water freed from these hazards by sterilization, boiling, adequate chlorination or filtration is essential. Such a drinking water supply also eliminates the necessity of entering the water of pools, lakes and irrigation channels in order to collect water for household purposes, and thus eliminates the risk of exposure to schistosome infection.

Provision of Safe Bathing Facilities

In hot climates the temptation to bathe can be well-nigh overwhelming, especially to children; and, since water is an important vehicle of infection, provision of pools with filtered and chlorinated water is an obvious but often neglected preventive measure.

Personal Prophylaxis

Many parasitic infections can be avoided by care and attention on the part of the individual. The adequate cooking of all meat, fish and shellfish; the washing or disinfection of salads or vegetables; the avoidance of food or drink from any doubtful or unclean source; the washing of hands before eating; the employment of repellent ointments; the wearing of protective clothing; and the use of nets and screens, are all measures which have been mentioned in the text and for which the responsibility rests with the individual.

Educational Propaganda

Although mentioned last, this measure is, perhaps, the most important, since the success of any measures taken to control a parasitic disease depend upon the co-operation of the population at hazard. In any major campaign against an endemic disease all the resources of modern publicity are brought into play via family, school and other groupings.

In conclusion, it may be mentioned that, since these infections recognise no national boundaries, international co-operation is essential in their control and elimination. This is now being achieved through the technical agencies of the United Nations, notably the World Health Organisation and the Food and Agriculture Organisation.

BIBLIOGRAPHY

Further information about the subjects discussed in this monograph may be found in the following works:

Belding, D. L. *Textbook of Clinical Parasitology*. New York. Appleton-Century-Crofts.

Brumpt, E. *Précis de Parasitologie*. Paris. Masson.

Craig, C. F. and Faust, E. C. *Clinical Parasitology*. Philadelphia. Lea and Febiger.

Herms, W. B. *Medical Entomology*. New York. Macmillan.

Hoare, C. A. *Medical Protozoology*. London. Baillière, Tindall and Cox.

Lapage, G. *Veterinary Parasitology*. London. Oliver and Boyd.

Mathieson, R. *Medical Entomology*. New York. Comstock.

Monnig, H. O. (revised Lapage, G.) *Veterinary Helminthology and Entomology*. London. Baillière, Tindall and Cox.

Watson, J. M. *Medical Helminthology*. London. Baillière, Tindall and Cox.

No suitable reference work on medical and veterinary malacology exists. The information about this subject is scattered through a vast range of articles in scientific journals and large monographs dealing with special groups of snails.

No editions or dates have been cited since these are all standard reference works of which new editions appear from time to time.

Chandler, A. C. *Introduction to Parasitology*. New York–London. Chapman and Hall.

This is the best book for the newcomer to parasitology. It is an eminently readable account of the principal parasites of man and domestic animals and the diseases which they cause.

The following large and detailed works provide admirable illustrations and a wealth of other information:

Morgan, B. B. and Hawkin, P. A. (1948). *Veterinary Protozoology*. Minneapolis. Burgess.

Morgan, B. B. and Hawkins, P. A. (1949). *Veterinary Helminthology*. Minneapolis. Burgess.

Neveu-Lemaire, M. (1943). *Traité de Protozoologie médicale et vétérinaire*. Paris. Vigot Frères.

Neveu-Lemaire, M. (1936). *Traité de Helminthologie médicale et vétérinaire*. Paris. Vigot Frères.

INDEX